THE CORONAVIRUS PREPAREDNESS HANDBOOK

How to Protect Your Home, School, Workplace, and Community from a Deadly Pandemic

TESS PENNINGTON,

BESTSELLING AUTHOR OF *THE PREPPER'S BLUEPRINT*

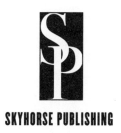

SKYHORSE PUBLISHING

Skyhorse Publishing books may be purchased in bulk at special discounts for sales promotion, corporate gifts, fund-raising, or educational purposes. Special editions can also be created to specifications. For details, contact the Special Sales Department, Skyhorse Publishing, 307 West 36th Street, 11th Floor, New York, NY 10018 or info@skyhorsepublishing.com.

Skyhorse® and Skyhorse Publishing® are registered trademarks of Skyhorse Publishing, Inc.®, a Delaware corporation.

Visit our website at www.skyhorsepublishing.com.

10 9 8 7 6 5 4 3 2 1

Library of Congress Cataloging-in-Publication Data is available on file.

Cover design by Mona Lin
Cover images: HardtIllustrations/Shutterstock.com and Getty Images

Print ISBN: 978-1-5107-6251-0

Printed in the United States of America

Contents

Responding to COVID-19 —
A Once-in-a-Century Pandemic?

By Bill Gates

First published in The New England Journal of Medicine, *Feb 28, 2020 Copyright © 2020, Massachusetts Medical Society, reprinted with permission*

In any crisis, leaders have two equally important responsibilities: solve the immediate problem and keep it from happening again. The Covid-19 pandemic is a case in point. We need to save lives now while also improving the way we respond to outbreaks in general. The first point is more pressing, but the second has crucial long-term consequences.

The long-term challenge — improving our ability to respond to outbreaks — isn't new. Global health experts have been saying for years that another pandemic whose speed and severity rivaled those of the 1918 influenza epidemic was a matter not of if but of when.[1] The Bill and Melinda Gates Foundation has committed substantial resources in recent years to helping the world prepare for such a scenario.

Now we also face an immediate crisis. In the past week, Covid-19 has started behaving a lot like the once-in-a-century pathogen we've been worried about. I hope it's not that bad, but we should assume it will be until we know otherwise.

There are two reasons that Covid-19 is such a threat. First, it can kill healthy adults in addition to elderly people with existing health problems. The data so far suggest that the virus has a case fatality risk around 1%; this rate would make it many times more severe than typical seasonal influenza, putting it somewhere between the 1957 influenza pandemic (0.6%) and the 1918 influenza pandemic (2%).[2]

Second, Covid-19 is transmitted quite efficiently. The average infected person spreads the disease to two or three others — an exponential rate of increase. There is also strong evidence that it can be transmitted by people who are just mildly ill or even presymptomatic.[3] That means Covid-19 will be much harder to contain than the Middle East respiratory syndrome or severe acute respiratory syndrome (SARS), which were spread much less efficiently and only by symptomatic people. In fact, Covid-19 has already caused 10 times as many cases as SARS in a quarter of the time.

National, state, and local governments and public health agencies can take steps over the next few weeks to slow the virus's spread. For example, in addition to helping their own citizens respond, donor governments can help low- and middle-income countries (LMICs) prepare for this pandemic.[4] Many LMIC health systems are already stretched thin, and a pathogen like the coronavirus can quickly overwhelm them. And poorer countries have little political or economic leverage, given wealthier countries' natural desire to put their own people first.

By helping African and South Asian countries get ready now, we can save lives and slow the global circulation of the virus. (A substantial portion of the commitment Melinda and I recently made to help kickstart the global response to Covid-19 — which could total up to $100 million — is focused on LMICs.)

The world also needs to accelerate work on treatments and vaccines for Covid-19.[5] Scientists sequenced the genome of the virus and developed several promising vaccine candidates in a matter of days, and the Coalition for Epidemic Preparedness Innovations is already preparing up to eight promising vaccine candidates for clinical trials. If some of these vaccines prove safe and effective in animal models, they could be ready for larger-scale trials as early as June. Drug discovery can also be accelerated by drawing on libraries of compounds that have already been tested for safety and by applying new screening techniques, including machine learning, to identify antivirals that could be ready for large-scale clinical trials within weeks.

All these steps would help address the current crisis. But we also need to make larger systemic changes so we can respond more efficiently and effectively when the next epidemic arrives.

It's essential to help LMICs strengthen their primary health care systems. When you build a health clinic, you're also creating part of the infrastructure for fighting epidemics. Trained health care workers not only deliver vaccines; they can also monitor disease patterns, serving as part of the early warning systems that alert the world to potential outbreaks.

We also need to invest in disease surveillance, including a case database that is instantly accessible to relevant organizations, and rules requiring countries to share information. Governments should have access to lists of trained personnel, from local leaders to global experts, who are prepared to deal with an epidemic immediately, as well as lists of supplies to be stockpiled or redirected in an emergency.

In addition, we need to build a system that can develop safe, effective vaccines and antivirals, get them approved, and deliver billions of doses within a few months after the discovery of a fast-moving pathogen. That's a tough challenge that presents technical, diplomatic, and budgetary obstacles, as well as demanding partnership between the public and private sectors. But all these obstacles can be overcome.

One of the main technical challenges for vaccines is to improve on the old ways of manufacturing proteins, which are too slow for responding to an epidemic. We need to develop platforms that are predictably safe, so regulatory reviews can happen quickly, and that make it easy for manufacturers to produce doses at low cost on a massive scale. For antivirals, we need an organized system to screen existing treatments and candidate molecules in a swift and standardized manner.

Another technical challenge involves constructs based on nucleic acids. These constructs can be produced within hours after a virus's genome has been sequenced; now we need to find ways to produce them at scale.

Beyond these technical solutions, we'll need diplomatic efforts to drive international collaboration and data sharing. Developing antivirals and vaccines involves massive clinical trials and licensing agreements that would cross national borders. We should make the most of global forums that can help achieve consensus on research priorities and trial protocols so that promising vaccine and antiviral candidates can move quickly through this process. These platforms include the World Health Organization R&D Blueprint, the International Severe Acute Respiratory and Emerging Infection Consortium trial network, and the Global Research Collaboration for Infectious Disease Preparedness. The goal of this work should be to get conclusive clinical trial results and regulatory approval in 3 months or less, without compromising patients' safety.

Then there's the question of funding. Budgets for these efforts need to be expanded several times over. Billions more dollars are needed to complete phase 3 trials and secure regulatory approval for coronavirus vaccines, and still more funding will be needed to improve disease surveillance and response.

Government funding is needed because pandemic products are extraordinarily high-risk investments; public funding will minimize risk for pharmaceutical companies and get them to jump in with both feet. In addition, governments and other donors will need to fund — as a global public good — manufacturing facilities that can generate a vaccine supply in a matter of weeks. These facilities can make vaccines for routine immunization programs in normal times and be quickly refitted for production during a pandemic. Finally, governments will need to finance the procurement and distribution of vaccines to the populations that need them.

Billions of dollars for antipandemic efforts is a lot of money. But that's the scale of investment required to solve the problem. And given the economic pain that an epidemic can impose — we're already seeing how Covid-19 can disrupt supply chains and stock markets, not to mention people's lives — it will be a bargain.

Finally, governments and industry will need to come to an agreement: during a pandemic, vaccines and antivirals can't simply be sold to the highest bidder. They should be available and affordable for people who are at the heart of the outbreak and in greatest need. Not only is such distribution the right thing to do, it's also the right strategy for short-circuiting transmission and preventing future pandemics.

These are the actions that leaders should be taking now. There is no time to waste.

1. Gates B. The next epidemic — lessons from Ebola. N Engl J Med 2015;372:1381-1384.
2. The Novel Coronavirus Pneumonia Emergency Response Epidemiology Team. The epidemiological characteristics of an outbreak of 2019 novel coronavirus disease (COVID-19) — China, 2020. China CDC Weekly 2020;2:1-10.
3. Hoehl S, Rabenau H, Berger A, et al. Evidence of SARS-CoV-2 infection in returning travelers from Wuhan, China. N Engl J Med. DOI: 10.1056/NEJMc2001899.
4. Frieden TR, Tappero JW, Dowell SF, et al. Safer countries through global health security. Lancet 2014;383:764-766.
5. Gates B. Innovation for pandemics. N Engl J Med 2018;378:2057-2060.

Introduction

On December 31, 2019, Chinese health officials reported a cluster of cases of acute respiratory illness in persons associated with the Hunan seafood and animal market in the city of Wuhan, Hubei Province, in central China.

In the days that followed, cases multiplied and overwhelmed the Chinese health care system, thus leading the Chinese government to take one of the most drastic attempts to control the viral spread in what has been dubbed as the "Wuhan Lockdown." This caused a frenzy of speculation and theories around the world when China locked down some of its highly populated cities. It would later be reported that Chinese officials intentionally withheld information that hospital workers had been infected by patients—a telltale sign of a contagion.

As the Chinese desperately tried to control the viral epicenter, it became clear that the virus was uncontained as countries outside of China began reported cases. On January 21, 2020, the first person in the United States with diagnosed 2019-nCoV infection was reported.

In late February, the first community spread case was confirmed in Santa Clara county, California. At this point in time, domestic spread and exposure to COVID-19 changed the game from mere containment and shined a light on the need to have more strategies in place for early detection and treatment.

Shortly following this, the CDC shifted strategies and began urging businesses, health-care facilities, and even schools to plan for ways to limit the impact of illness when it spreads in the community.

What can be amassed from leading health experts is they are at a loss on how to contain this new, highly contagious virus. In the words of Tedros Adhanom Ghebreyesus, Director-General of the World Health Organization (WHO), "We are in uncharted territory with COVID-19. We have never before seen a respiratory pathogen that is capable of community transmission, but which can also be contained with the right measures."[1]

As the world sits on the eve of a new pandemic, many wonder how it has come to this. Like all viruses, the coronavirus, in general, is intelligent, and its evolving nature makes it more of an enigma due to its ability to mutate and survive. Viruses have threatened the health of animal and human populations for centuries, and as sophisticated as our medical system is these days, we still have not been able to develop both a universal vaccine and highly effective antiviral drugs.

COVID-19 is a rapidly evolving situation, and health experts globally are trying to find the answers to the vital questions of how, from an epidemiological level, this "killer flu" has the capacity to cause so much disaster to humans. After 100 years of viral study, scientists still do not understand how many viruses work, what the proteins in the virus do, how they interact with one another, how they interact with host cells. Even the simplest of questions surrounding virology may go unanswered. This is both frustrating and intriguing that such a microscopic thing can elude some of the brightest minds. It is every virialogists hope to find these answers and hopefully, find a cure.

While quarantines, travel restrictions, and increased coronavirus screenings for those entering and exiting the country help reduce the spread of COVID-19, many believe it is simply too little too late. And, while it is too early to tell, speculation is circulating that the coronavirus was in the United States out in the open weeks before authorities came to the realization. Now that the contagion is out there, there is no denying that it is time to take the appropriate steps needed to keep your family healthy and safe.

How This Book Will Help

You may have purchased this book in response to the initial wave of COVID-19 hitting the world. Many may think it is too late to prepare because it is already spread or seems to have been contained. What you may not realize is that experts say the second wave may be coming, and unless we have a vaccine when it hits, it could be significantly farther reaching than the first.

This book goes beyond basic handwashing and social distancing protocols suggested by the CDC. This book will explain the strategies that the CDC is using to measure the progression of the disease. We will look at historic pandemics and learn from them in order to help your family stay ahead of what is to come and help you develop a personalized preparedness plan that can be implemented quickly. The best piece of advice this author can give you is to start preparing now before the panic ensues. Critical items for living like food, water, medicine, and sanitation items will quickly disappear in a pandemic emergency and shortages could last for the duration of the event.

As well, and perhaps, most importantly, even though health officials are saying the concern is low for this novel virus, what is happening in parts of the world say otherwise. Now is the time to prepare for the likelihood of outbreaks affecting your daily lives including social distancing protocols for local commerce, business, and distance-learning for schools. It is important to know what we are facing in terms of lifestyle changes, economic turmoil, and ultimately, how to keep our families healthy. It is a global concern that a quick-moving pathogen has the potential to kill tens of millions of people, disrupt economies, and destabilize national security. And as we have seen throughout history, though COVID-19 will eventually pass, viruses in general will never go away. They will only continue to find ways to infect and spread. Just as our will is to survive, so is theirs.

CHAPTER 1

Just the Facts

At the onset of the virus, here's what we know: the 2019 Novel Coronavirus, or 2019-nCoV, is a new respiratory virus first identified in Wuhan, Hubei Province, China in late 2019. This virus is deadly, highly contagious, and spreading rapidly. It is also considered a novel virus, meaning that it has not been previously identified and is not the same as other coronaviruses that commonly circulate among humans and cause mild illness, like the common cold.

Seven strains of coronavirus are known to infect humans, including this new virus, causing illnesses in the respiratory tract. Four of those strains cause common colds. Two others, by contrast, rank among the deadliest of human infections: severe acute respiratory syndrome, or SARS, and Middle East Respiratory Syndrome, or MERS. The medical consensus is the COVID-19 virus is less deadly than SARS. However, it is more transmissible; the human-to-human transmission of COVID-19 is higher than SARS. The thing you need to know is this: the virus itself is lung specific and only has cell receptors for lung cells. Therefore, it *only* infects your lungs. The only way for the virus to infect you is through infected droplets from coughs and sneezes that enter through your nose or mouth or eyes via your hands.

Origin of Coronavirus

Because this is such a large category of viruses, it's difficult to tell where it came from. Some say it jumped from animals to humans, but researchers have so far failed to produce conclusive evidence to support that hypothesis, although it does make sense. Many viruses have adapted and mutated to jump to humans in the past, causing immense harm to humanity (think AIDS/HIV which scientists say "officially" came from monkeys). This virus probably originally emerged from an animal source but now seems to be spreading from person to person, according to the Centers for Disease Control and Prevention.

It is also unclear whether this novel virus is seasonal or longer lasting. Because this is a rapidly changing event, only time will tell.

The World Health Organization has a six-stage influenza program that explains how viruses jump from animals to humans:

Stage 1: No animal influenza virus circulating among animals has been reported to cause infection in humans.

Stage 2: An animal influenza virus circulating in domesticated or wild animals is known to have caused infection in humans and is therefore considered a specific potential pandemic threat.

Stage 3: An animal or human-animal influenza reassortant virus has caused sporadic cases or small clusters of disease in people, but it has not resulted in human-to-human transmission sufficient to sustain community-level outbreaks.

Stage 4: Human-to-human transmission of an animal or human-animal influenza reassortant virus able to sustain community-level outbreaks has been verified.

Stage 5: The same identified virus has caused sustained community level outbreaks in two or more countries in one WHO region.

Stage 6: In addition to the criteria defined in Stage 5, the same virus has caused sustained community level outbreaks in at least one other country in another WHO region.

Post-peak period: Levels of pandemic influenza in most countries with adequate surveillance have dropped below peak levels.

Post-pandemic period: Levels of influenza activity have returned to the levels seen for seasonal influenza in most countries with adequate surveillance.

How Do You Catch the Coronavirus?

While our understanding of this virus continues to evolve, we know that coronaviruses, in general, are spread in the same manner as the common cold—through infected water droplets from a sneeze, cough, or the breath. Because the coronavirus is novel, the human population has little or no immunity against it. This allows the virus to spread quickly from person to person worldwide.

It's important to note that person-to-person spread can happen on a continuum (meaning just because you have had the virus, that doesn't mean you won't get it again). If these droplets come in contact with the eyes, nose, or mouth of an individual directly or indirectly, the individual may become infected. Health experts agree that a person can get COVID-19 by touching a surface or object that has the virus on it and then touching their own mouth, nose, or possibly their eyes, but this is not thought to be the main way the virus spreads.

It is uncertain how long the virus that causes COVID-19 survives on surfaces, but it seems to behave like other coronaviruses. Studies suggest that coronaviruses (including preliminary information on the COVID-19 virus) may persist on surfaces for a few hours or up to several days. This may vary under different conditions (e.g. type of surface, temperature or humidity of the environment, etc.).

According to the CDC, the virus is thought to be spread mainly person-to-person in the following ways:

- Between people who are in close contact with one another (within about 6 feet).

- Through respiratory droplets produced when an infected person coughs or sneezes. These droplets can land in the mouths or noses of people who are nearby or possibly be inhaled into the lungs.
- From contact with infected surfaces or objects.

Soft surfaces like fabrics and carpet are not reported to be of concern for the presence of coronavirus. What health officials are concerned with are frequently touched items. Unfortunately, there isn't a lot you can do to make a dent in all of those nasty germs stuck on surfaces in public places like grocery store cars, park benches, school desks, and even at the airport. But you can encourage your children to wash their hands frequently and keep their hands away from their little faces. But at home, there are some surfaces more prone to being carriers of germs and illnesses. These areas in the home include tabletops, countertops, remote controls, game controllers, computer keyboards, doorknobs, sinks, light switches, faucet handles, sinks, countertop, tub, and toilet (including the entire seat and the toilet handle).

What Coronavirus Is Not and the Misinformation Surrounding COVID-19

The worst types of disasters are the ones that we do not know much about. This, of course, invites speculation, hysteria, and anxiety-driven decisions, and ultimately clouds what the facts really are. What is clear is that when a contagious disease is breaking out in random parts of a nation and people are dying from it, it frightens people. As a result, people are going to want answers; they are going to want to protect their families, and they will look to the country's leaders for guidance. Practical advice and truth must be shared in order to prevent misinformation from running rampant and the "chicken little effect" from taking over.

Here are some common questions surrounding the novel COVID-19:

- **Is COVID-19 airborne?** There has been some confusion on whether or not the virus is airborne, such as in the diseases of the measles or chicken pox. According to the CDC, no evidence suggests that this virus is airborne. However, if you are sick, it is highly recommended that you protect others around you and in your community by wearing a mask to prevent the spread of germs from coughs and sneezes.

- **Who is the most at risk?** Moreover, individuals who are over 60 years old or have an underlying health condition such as cardiovascular disease, have a weakened immune system, a respiratory condition, or diabetes could have a high risk of developing a severe form of the virus. In a published study in the official China CDC Weekly, it was revealed that out of a subset of 44,700 infections confirmed in Chinese patients through lab tests, more than 80 percent were at least 60 years old, with half over 70.

- **Is it safe to receive packages in the mail?** Yes. The likelihood of an infected person contaminating commercial goods is low, and the risk of catching the virus that causes COVID-19 from a package that has been moved, travelled, and exposed to different conditions and temperature is also low.

- **Can I catch COVID-19 from my pet?** No. There is no evidence that companion animals or pets such as cats and dogs have been infected or could spread the virus that causes COVID-19.

- **Will warm weather stop the outbreak?** It is not yet known whether weather and temperature will impact the spread of COVID-19. Some other viruses, like the common cold and flu, spread more during cold weather months, but that does not mean it is impossible to become sick with these viruses during other months. At this time, it is not known whether the spread of

COVID-19 will decrease when weather becomes warmer. There is much more to learn about the transmissibility, severity, and other features associated with COVID-19 and investigations are ongoing.

- **Are pregnant women and children more susceptible to getting COVID-19?** There is not currently information from published scientific reports about susceptibility of pregnant women to COVID-19. Pregnant women experience immunologic and physiologic changes that might make them more susceptible to viral respiratory infections, including COVID-19. There is no evidence that children are more susceptible to COVID-19. In fact, most confirmed cases of COVID-19 reported from China have occurred in adults. Relatively few infections in children have been reported, including in very young children.
- **Should I be tested for COVID-19?** Call your healthcare professional if you feel sick with fever, cough, or difficulty breathing and have been in close contact with a person known to have COVID-19, or if you live in or have recently traveled from an area with ongoing spread of COVID-19.

Symptoms of the Coronavirus

COVID-19 can be difficult to diagnose based on symptoms because it presents so similarly to a general cold or flu. Reported illnesses have ranged from mild symptoms to severe illness and death for confirmed coronavirus disease 2019 (COVID-19) cases.

Symptoms may appear 2–14 days after exposure:

- Fever
- Cough
- Shortness of breath
- Pneumonia (in some cases)
- Body aches

- Nausea and/or vomiting
- Diarrhea

What Exactly Does COVID-19 Do to a Person?

The virus infects the lower respiratory tract and multiplies. It attacks two specific lung cells: mucus producing cells (protecting lungs from pathogens) and ciliated cells (clears debris, including viruses, out of the lungs). Ciliated cells are thought to be the preferred cells that the coronavirus attacks. When the cells are attacked and die, they slough out into the lungs, which fill with debris and fluid. Many patients infected with this virus end up getting pneumonia as a result.

The immune system responds to the lungs and, as a result, the lungs become inflamed. While this inflammation is a normal part of fighting infection, in the lungs it can be uncomfortable. In some cases where the immune system is fighting the coronavirus there is a hyper-reactivity of the immune system which results in more healthy tissue dying off in the lungs and worsening the pneumonia.

The inflammation also results in more permeable alveoli, the tiny air sacs in the lungs, filling with fluid and crowding out air so that not enough oxygen can reach the bloodstream. In severe cases, it floods the lungs so a person can no longer breathe. The damage can also cause a cytokine storm, which can result in multi-organ failure. More on this in Chapter 2.

As damage to the lungs increases, pulmonary destruction escalates quickly. Patients who get to this stage in the coronavirus could incur permanent lung damage in the form of scars that stiffen the lungs, or they may die.

As frightening as this sounds, most people only become mildly ill, or are infected but are asymptomatic, while others show mild symptoms for a few days and then it quickly escalates into more severe symptoms of pneumonia and organ failure. It should be noted that a person who is asymptomatic may be recovering from the virus and still make others ill. It's not clear how often asymptomatic transmission is occurring. The antibodies produced from this particular virus are weak and often do not provide any immunity to further infections.

Illness due to COVID-19 infection is generally mild, especially for children and young adults. However, it can cause serious illness: about 1 in every 5 people who catch it need hospital care.

Dr. Maria Van Kerkhove, who heads the WHO's Health Emergencies Program, warns, "You have mild cases, which look like the common cold, which have some respiratory symptoms, sore throat, runny nose, fever, all the way through pneumonia. And there can be varying levels of severity of pneumonia all the way through multi-organ failure and death," she told reporters in Geneva on February 7.

> Incidentally, in the Journal of the American Medical Association (JAMA) on February 7 reported that "the most common symptoms were fever, fatigue and dry cough. A third of the patients also reported muscle pain and difficulty breathing, while about 10 percent had atypical symptoms, including diarrhoea and nausea."
>
> The patients, who ranged in age from 22 to 92, were admitted to the Zhongnan Hospital of Wuhan University between January 1 and 28. "The median age of patients is between 49 and 56 years," JAMA said. "Cases in children have been rare."[2]

Patients are thought to be most contagious when they are symptomatic. However, there have been reports that found an asymptomatic person who transmitted COVID-19 to 5 other people and may have had a longer incubation time of 19 days.

Emergency symptoms for CHILDREN:
- Fast breathing or trouble breathing
- Bluish skin color

- Not drinking enough fluids
- Not waking up or not interacting
- Being so irritable that the child does not want to be held
- Fever with a rash
- Flu-like symptoms that improve but then return with a fever and a worse cough

Emergency symptoms for ADULTS:

- Difficulty breathing or shortness of breath
- Pain or pressure in the chest or abdomen
- Sudden dizziness
- Confusion
- Severe or persistent vomiting
- Flu-like symptoms that improve but then return with a fever and a worse cough

*Additional emergency signs for infants include being unable to eat, no tears when crying, and significantly fewer wet diapers than normal.

Mortality Rate and Morbidity Rate: Why Are They So Important?

To further understand this novel virus, it is important to understand the mortality rate, what it is, and why it is measured. Mortality and morbidity rates are important tools of indication of the health status of a population. In simple terms, the underlying difference between morbidity and mortality rates are life and death.

- **Morbidity Rate** is the state of being symptomatic or unhealthy from a disease or condition. This is important to measure because in the investigation of a deadly pathogen it helps tell the story and provides patterns of occurrence of illness. Further, indicators of morbidity such as the prevalence of chronic diseases and disabilities become more important in tracking.

- **Mortality Rate** is related to the number of deaths caused by the health event under investigation. In high mortality settings, information on trends of death (by causes) help to substantiate the progress of health programs.

Pandemics, in general, can cause significant, widespread increases in morbidity and mortality and have disproportionately higher mortality impacts. With regards to COVID-19, early estimates had the mortality rate between 2% and about 3.4%, according to calculations of confirmed cases and deaths worldwide.

It is alarming when you read a 3.4% mortality rate, but you have to understand that when you see this mortality rate, it is not 100% accurate. Real time numbers are inaccurate right now because different countries can be better or worse at spotting the milder, harder to count cases. As well, there is an issue with under-reported cases or cases not reported at all because the symptoms may be so mild that the infected patient does not realize they have it.

It is easy to overestimate the death rate. But you can also get it wrong in the other direction. Scientists cannot study the morbidity rate if a person with the mild version of the illness does not go to a doctor to have it diagnosed. As the data evolves, scientists will develop a clearer picture of who will be most at risk if the coronavirus outbreak continues to spread into more communities.

Viral Mutations

It is not uncommon for viruses to mutate and change after they jump from animals to humans. After all, a pathogen's job is to evade the immune system, create more copies of itself, and spread to other hosts.

A virus's ability to drift from its original form makes it difficult for vaccines to work and a body's natural immunity to keep up and prepare. As well, it makes the job of health officials all the more difficult because it is harder to track and treat infected patients. Moreover, there is a possibility that those who have recovered from the initial viral outbreak can become re-infected.

It is believed that we may not develop a natural immunity to COVID-19, but only time will tell. And while the latest research at the time of this writing is that COVID-19 may continue to infect people due to lack of immunity, humans have developed an immunity to other viruses studied. Hopefully, in time, this will be the case with COVID-19.

As an example, consider the flu. According to a report from the Neiman Foundation for the *Harvard Journal*, "Like all living things, influenza makes small errors—mutations—when it copies its genetic code during reproduction. But influenza lacks the ability to repair those errors, because it is an RNA virus; RNA, unlike DNA, lacks a self-correcting mechanism. As a result, influenza is not genetically stable."[3]

A study from Nankai University in Tianjin lead by Professor Ruan Jishou discovered that the new SARS-Cov-2 coronavirus that causes the COVID-19 disease has a mutated gene that is found in the HIV virus. As a result, the study found two distinct versions of the virus, which they named L and S.

L Strain – This is the more aggressive and faster-spreading strain, compared to its milder counterpart, S. This strain is responsible for around 70% of infected patients. Due to its aggressive nature, it has become less common as the outbreak has gone on, with it apparently struggling to spread since early January. The L strain surged at the beginning of the outbreak and made people so ill, those who caught it were quickly diagnosed and isolated. This isolation has given it less opportunity to spread widely. Experts suggest the "human intervention" and lockdown of areas where it was spreading fast is controlling the transmission rate, and hopefully leading to this virus strain to burn itself out.

S Strain – This milder strain is less severe but people will carry it for longer before ending up in a hospital, thus spreading the infection to more people. This is the original strain and, from an evolutionary standpoint, this strain is winning out compared to its more aggressive form.[4]

Jishou states, "This finding suggests that 2019-nCoV coronavirus may be significantly different from the SARS coronavirus in the infection pathway and has the added potency of using the packing mechanisms of other viruses such as HIV."

That added potency, the study revealed, was a mutation that can generate a structure known as a cleavage site (similar to those in HIV and Ebola) in the new coronavirus's spike protein. The cleavage site structure's role is to trick the human furin protein, so it will cut and activate the spike protein and cause a "direct fusion" of the viral and cellular membranes.

Because viruses are part of the RNA family, mutations in viral diseases are normal. It is still out for debate about which coronavirus strain will win out in this pandemic, but the bright side to all of this is scientists are one step closer to understanding the virus and, hopefully, finding a way to bring an end to its spread.

Recovery Times

If you or a loved one contracts COVID-19, it is important to understand what the recovery times will look like. While recovery times vary, the sliver of good news is, it seems that most people who get sick *will* recover from COVID-19.

- In non-severe cases, the recovery may be similar to the aftermath of a flu-like illness, and those with mild symptoms may recover within a few days.
- In moderate cases, which may or may not have the presence of pneumonia, recovery may take longer (days to weeks).
- Twenty percent of cases may be severe and/or life-threatening and could take months for a person to recover, or the person may die.

Most people who fall ill recover within two weeks. People with more severe cases generally recover in three to six weeks. During the recovery period, it is important to do what you can to help your body recover. Your body needs time and energy to fight off the virus, which means that your daily routine should be put on the backburner. Stay home until you can be tested to make sure you are no longer contagious, hydrate, get plenty of sleep, eat healthy foods, and allow your body the time it needs to heal.

Do not be alarmed if after you begin to recover from this serious viral illness that you may feel symptoms similar to depression. There is a condition called post-viral depression, something that many who recovered from the Spanish Flu admitted to experiencing.

Almost any viral infection can trigger post-viral syndrome because when a virus enters the body, it causes the immune system to respond and attack. This response can put stress on the body and cause inflammation. The effects of this response often leave people feeling down, fatigued, and sometimes depressed. Some symptoms include:

- confusion
- trouble concentrating
- headaches
- aches and pains in the muscles
- stiff joints

- a sore throat
- swollen lymph nodes

If you are experiencing any of these symptoms after recovery, the most important thing to do is talk to your doctor and let them know. As well, this is your body's way of telling you to slow down and let it rest.

Which Is Deadlier: The Flu Or Coronavirus?

The coronavirus is novel, meaning it has not been seen before. A flu pandemic occurs when a new flu virus that is different from seasonal flu viruses emerges and spreads quickly between people, causing illness worldwide. Most people will lack immunity to the pandemic flu virus. Pandemic flu can be more severe, causing more deaths than seasonal flu. Because it is a new virus, a vaccine may not be available right away. A pandemic could therefore overwhelm normal operations in schools, workplaces, and other community settings.

While the typical flu causes more harm every year, at this point, coronavirus seems to be more deadly when compared with the average flu strands. On average, seasonal flu strains kill 0.1% of people who become infected from it. At the time of writing this, the mortality rate for coronavirus is around 1.4% – 2%. Even if it dropped to 1%, it still is 10 times more lethal than the standard influenza that we have on a seasonal basis.

The new coronavirus also seems to be more contagious than most flu strains. The infection rate of the coronavirus is averaging to about 2.2, but this number may not be exact. Due to some coronavirus cases having mild symptoms in patients, it is hard to access accurate numbers, because some patients may not realize they have the virus.

In both the flu and the illnesses caused by the coronavirus, people may be contagious before symptoms develop, making it next to impossible to control the spread of the virus.

Interestingly, the average flu seems to be more dangerous to children. If a child becomes infected with the coronavirus, on average, their symptoms seem to be mild.

What the Princess Cruises Can Teach Us About COVID-19

Cruise ships are notorious for spreading illnesses. The Diamond Princess and Grand Princess cruise ships exposed thousands of their passengers to the coronavirus. This is the timeline of the nightmarish month at sea on the Diamond Princess as recorded by the Princess Cruise line.

February 1, 2020 - Princess Cruises confirms that a guest onboard tested positive for coronavirus on February 1. The passenger traveled for 5 days on board Diamond Princess from Yokohama, Tokyo and disembarked on January 25th in Tokyo, Japan. He visited a local Hong Kong hospital, six days after leaving the ship, where he later tested positive for coronavirus on February 1. According to the ship logs, during the voyage, the passenger was not seen in the ship medical center for any reported illnesses. The guest is currently admitted to a local hospital and reported to be in a stable condition.

February 4, 2020 – Princess Cruises confirms that Diamond Princess has a 24-hour delay to allow Japan public health authorities to check the health status of all guests and crew on board.

Later that day, Princess Cruises decided to cancel the next voyage of Diamond Princess to help facilitate the health screening and records review process after testing found that 10 people on board tested positive for Coronavirus. This includes two Australian guests, three Japanese guests, three guests from Hong Kong, and one guest from the U.S. in addition to one Filipino crewmember.

The infected passengers were taken ashore by Japanese Coast Guard and transported to local hospitals for care. For the remaining passengers and crew, the ship will remain under quarantine in Yokohama for the length of the quarantine (at least 14 days) as required by the Ministry of Health.

The ship plans to go out to sea to perform normal marine operations including, but not limited to, the

February 6, 2020 - New Cases / Nationalities / Quarantine End Date: New cases arise onboard Diamond Princess. According to ship logs, 41 people tested positive. The Japanese Ministry of Health has confirmed this is the last batch to be tested and the quarantine end date will be February 19, unless there are any other unforeseen developments.

February 9, 2020 - Additional Cases Confirmed by Ministry of Health: 66 confirmed cases of coronavirus are now confirmed onboard Diamond Princess.

February 12, 2020 - A voluntary "phased approach" disembarkation of guests has been planned for those who completed their quarantine period at a shoreside facility. The first to disembark will be the most medically vulnerable guests, including older adults with pre-existing health conditions.

Guests in the first phase will be tested for coronavirus. If the test is positive, they will be transported to a local hospital for further evaluation and isolation. If the test is negative, they will be given the option to leave the ship and be transported to a quarantine housing facility.

February 16, 2020 - The Japanese Ministry of Health states there are 67 new positive cases of COVID-19 onboard Diamond Princess.

February 18, 2020 - The total number of new positive cases onboard Diamond Princess is now at a staggering 169. As a result, the cruise ship was denied entry into a San Francisco port due to 20 coronavirus cases among 3,500 people on board.

February 19, 2020 - Embassies of countries including Canada, Australia and Hong Kong are coordinating the collection and transport of their respective citizens (guests and crew) via charter flights. Citizens will be required to have an additional 14 days of quarantine upon arrival in their country of origin.

A negative COVID-19 test following this quarantine will be required before being allowed to travel to their final destination.

February 20, 2020 - Approximately six hundred guests onboard Diamond Princess were the first to be cleared by the Japanese Ministry of Health and released to disembark the ship yesterday.

February 27, 2020 - All guests have disembarked the Diamond Princess. There are fewer than 500 team members on board, with some awaiting government charter flights. Princess Cruises has hired a WHO-certified company to provide team members with health and wellbeing care during a quarantine at a land-based center in Japan.

But the journey did not end there for everyone. Quarantined at sea, the cruise line had been forbidden to dock in San Francisco amid evidence that the vessel was the breeding ground for a cluster of nearly 20 cases that resulted in at least one death after its previous voyage.

On March 5, 2020, docked 45 miles off the California coast, the National Guard dropped coronavirus testing kits on board in order to test the passengers to ensure they were safe to dock on US soil. Out of the 44 remaining passengers and crew, 21 tested positive for the virus including 19 crew members. While the cruise line has been accepted to unboard at an Oakland port, extra precautions are being made to ensure the passengers and crew do not have COVID-19 and will further spread the contagion to the surrounding communities. At least 21 of the nearly 3,000 people who subsequently took the same ship to Hawaii have tested positive for the virus. All of those passengers remain on board, and many more still need to be tested. It's unclear what will happen to those who are found to be sick.

Dr. Grant Tarling, the cruise's medical officer, said the man who died at Kaiser Permanente Roseville Medical Center after leaving the ship sought onboard medical care Feb. 20 and had been sick for several days. Tarling said two waiters who served the man multiple times were subsequently infected.

Incidentally, Princess Cruises also owns the Diamond Princess, another ship that was quarantined in Yokohama, Japan, and experienced a coronavirus outbreak that infected more than 700 passengers.

Without realizing it, the 3,500 passengers unknowingly became the perfect test study for understanding the virus in a closed off environment. The passengers who were quarantined off the coast of the United States may have helped experts better understand the virus and it effects.

While COVID-19 is not considered airborne, it is easily transmissible from the moisture droplets from coughs. The ventilation systems on board the cruise ship, which were all inter-connected, likely played into the transmission rate. As well, because some of the rooms in the cruise ships do not have access to fresh air and provide poorer air quality, the virus likely festered and spread more easily.

Health experts have warned about the potential for cruise ship outbreaks for years. Purdue University's Qingyan Chen, an expert on ventilation during virus outbreaks, weighs in on the subject.

> A ship's ventilation system, which relies on recirculated air filtered by medium-strength air filters, is an efficient way of spreading virus particles from room to room aboard a ship, said Chen. In a 2015 study, he and his colleagues looked at the spread of flu aboard cruise ships, finding that one infected person would typically lead to more than 40 cases a week later on a 2,000 passenger cruise, with transmission occurring through the ventilation system. In contrast, on land, the coronavirus seems to have a reproductive rate of two new cases per infected person, which would lead to three new cases in that time.[5]

Breakdowns and gaps in necessary protocols were also exposed. While it is unknown if one of the passengers who is thought be the one who brought the virus onboard knew he was infected or if the symptoms came on after boarding, this has taught cruise ships to have better boarding protocols, which now include:

- Further enhancement of entry and exit screening and shipboard testing for the coronavirus.
- New quarantine standards coordinated with the CDC for all cruise ships.
- A protocol to move any patients that contract the coronavirus or otherwise become seriously ill to land-based facilities.

Also, even though the cruise ship took the necessary precautions and quarantined passengers, crew members who unknowingly were infected with the virus came to the rooms to deliver meals and inadvertently exposed more passengers to the deadly virus.

At this point, the unknowns of this health crisis seem to outweigh the knowns. And until a vaccine is found—which is months if not years away—the only way to prevent it is to avoid it.

CHAPTER 2

Pandemics: What Are They and What Can We Expect?

"Everyone knows that pestilences have a way of reoccurring in the world; yet somehow we find it hard to believe in ones that crash down on our hads from a blue sky. There have been as many plagues as wars in history; yet always plagues and wars take people equally by surprise."
—Albert Camus, *The Plague*

What Are Pandemics?

The word "pandemic" comes from the Greek word *pandemos*, which means "everybody." "Pan," meaning everyone, "demos," meaning population. Pandemics do not discriminate between the rich and the poor or which political affiliation you side with. They are unrelenting and have the ability to create a pivotal life moment. These large-scale outbreaks of infectious disease can greatly increase morbidity and mortality over a wide geographic area and cause significant economic, social, and political disruption.

A pandemic is not a solitary event. The event accelerates and decelerates and repeats itself. If the conditions are right, there are waves of activity in pandemics.

Pandemics can cause significant, widespread increases in morbidity and mortality and have disproportionately higher mortality impacts on LMICs (lower and middle income countries).

- Pandemics can cause economic damage through multiple channels, including short-term fiscal shocks and longer-term negative shocks to economic growth.
- Individual behavioral changes, such as fear-induced aversion to workplaces and other public gathering places, are a primary cause of negative shocks to economic growth during pandemics.
- Some pandemic mitigation measures can cause significant social and economic disruption.
- The death toll in a pandemic is generally higher than that in an epidemic.
- In countries with weak institutions and legacies of political instability, pandemics can increase political stresses and tensions. In these contexts, outbreak response measures such as quarantines have sparked violence and tension between states and citizens.

It is important to understand what we are facing, what strategies the CDC is undertaking to contain and prepare for more community-spread cases, and ultimately, how you can survive it. As well, there are some things we can learn from past pandemic events in order to help us with our present reality. After all, the best way to prepare for this type of event is to understand what it is, learn from it, and make an informed preparedness plan with the facts. Let's start with some essential terminology and move forward.

What Is an Epidemic?

A disease is called an epidemic when it spreads to multiple communities. It is often a sudden increase in the number of cases of a disease above what is normally expected in that population in that area. As an epidemic comes under control, health officials will be able to decide what the reproduction number is; that is, the rate of infection.

What Is a Cluster?

"Cluster" refers to an aggregation of cases grouped in place and time that are suspected to be greater than the number expected, even though the expected number may not be known. For example, the coronavirus outbreaks in Santa Clara county are a cluster of cases.

What Is an Outbreak?

"Outbreak" carries the same definition of epidemic but is often used for a more limited geographic area. According to the CDC, an outbreak attacks many peoples at about the same time and may spread through one or several communities. Outbreaks can range from food poisoning to enterovirus to seasonal flu. In the last two years, CDC has sent scientists and doctors out more than 750 times to respond to health threats due to outbreaks.

What Is a Pandemic?

A "pandemic" is an epidemic of disease that has spread across a large region, for instance multiple continents, or worldwide. Pandemics are naturally reoccurring disasters that tend to occur suddenly and without warning. It is important to note the CDC investigates new contagious diseases—averaging one new contagion per year. These contagious diseases can emerge right here or, as we are currently witnessing, are only a plane-ride away. Because pandemics are fast moving, without a vaccination on hand, there could be the potential for catastrophic death rates.

What Is a Cytokine Storm?

Cytokines are a diverse group of small proteins specific to the immune system that are secreted by cells for the purpose of intercellular signaling and communication. Cytokines essentially mediate and regulate immunity, inflammation, and hematopoiesis.

When an infection is severe, cytokine production can grow out of control, causing a "cytokine storm," an immune response where an overproduction of immune cells will occur. In the case of a flu infection, a surge of activated immune cells go into the lungs causing large-scale inflammation in the body. Blood vessels become more permeable and fluid seeps out making it more difficult for blood and oxygen to reach the rest of the body. This has the potential to cause damage to organs, especially the lungs and kidneys, and even lead to death. This was seen in many cases during the Spanish Flu Pandemic.

The primary symptoms of a cytokine storm are high fever, swelling and redness, extreme fatigue, and nausea. In some cases, the immune reaction may be fatal due to extensive damage to the lungs with severe hemorrhaging.

What We Can Learn from Historical Pandemics

It's natural to be fearful when it comes to the possibility of a world-spread contagion. Afterall, any stories about pestilence are full of suffering and death. Perhaps the most popular pandemic is one learned in the history books. The bubonic plague, or the Black Death, ravaged Europe and Asia and it took over 200 years for Europe to get its population back to where it was before the disease.

It is important to learn from history, and some things we can glean from past pandemic events help us with what we may be facing in the near future. The great plague that occurred in Athens in 430 B.C., and which was described by Thucydides, was probably caused by a pandemic influenza virus. In more recent history, there was the cholera epidemic that occurred during the period of 1899–1923, the Asian flu that occurred in 1957 and killed 2 million people, as well as the 1968 Hong Kong flu that killed over a million people.

Some other notable pandemics were:

Bubonic Plague: Peaking in the mid 1300s, the Black Death or bubonic plague likely occurred from the disease being transmitted from rodents to humans by the bite of infected fleas.

The plague is believed to have started in China along the trade routes to the West. Although it was relatively well contained in the Isles, it became an even greater threat to the world when the virus became airborne and quickly spread from human to human. Occurring throughout Eurasia, it is estimated to have killed 30–60 percent of Europe's population or roughly 75–200 million people.

One of the possible theories regarding what ended the bubonic plague is that it was better personal hygiene practices, cremations rather than burials, and the implementation of quarantines. Somehow, those who were uninfected quickly learned to remain in their homes and only leave when absolutely necessary. Moreover, many people left population-dense areas to ride out the bubonic plague in the country.

The Spanish Flu: One of the more deadly pandemics on record occurred 100 years ago. The Spanish Flu of 1918 caused a global pandemic that was so devastating that it infected an estimated one-third of the planet's population and killed an estimated 20 million to 50 million victims, and the average life expectancy was reduced by 13 years.

In the first wave of this pandemic, the new strain of an influenza virus hit military camps in Europe during World War I. Both sides were affected by this virus, but that was only the beginning. The first wave was mild in comparison to when the second wave hit. Months later, the bigger, much deadlier second wave hit and swept across the globe.

Incidentally, this was the last time the US used enforced large-scale isolation and quarantine efforts.

This naturally occurring pandemic was during a time when global travel was not readily available, accessible highways and/or transportation systems were at a minimum, and there were not as many mega-cities. In the case of the Spanish Flu, there were three pandemic waves, the second being the most fatal.

The Spanish flu hit different age groups, displaying a so-called "W-trend", with infections typically peaking in children and the elderly, with an intermediate spike in healthy young adults. In these last cases, lack of pre-existing virus-specific and/or cross-reactive antibodies and cellular immunity probably contributed to the high attack rate and rapid spread of the 1918 H1N1 virus, and to that "cytokine storm" which ultimately destroyed the lungs.

The Swine Flu: In the spring of 2009, a novel influenza A (H1N1) virus emerged. Dubbed "The Swine Flu" because in the past, the people who caught it had direct contact with pigs.

Swine Flu was first detected in the US and spread quickly across the country and the world. Between April 12, 2009 and April 10, 2010, there were 60.8 million cases reported, 274,304 hospitalizations, and 12,469 deaths due to the virus. The CDC estimates 575,400 people died worldwide.

Though the 2009 flu pandemic primarily affected children and young and middle-aged adults, the impact of the (H1N1) pdm09 virus on the global population during the first year was less severe than that of previous pandemics. It has now become a regular part of influenza planning and circulates seasonally in the US, still causing significant illness, hospitalizations, and deaths.

How The CDC Measures Pandemic Events

There are two main factors that can be used to determine the impact of a pandemic. The first is clinical severity, or how serious the illness is. The second factor is transmissibility, or how easily the pandemic virus spreads from person to person. These two factors combined are used to guide decisions about which actions CDC recommends at a given time during the pandemic.

Pandemic Waves and Measuring Disease Progression

Many pandemics are characterized by multiple waves of activity during the pandemic period. Multiple pandemic waves of illness are likely to occur with each wave lasting 2 to 3 months.

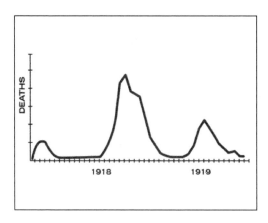

In the Spanish Flu Pandemic of 1918, there were three different waves of illness during the pandemic, starting in March 1918 and subsiding by summer of 1919. The pandemic peaked in the US during the second wave, in the fall of 1918. This highly fatal second wave was responsible for most of the US deaths attributed to the pandemic.

Historically speaking, the largest waves have occurred in the fall and winter, but the seasonality of a pandemic cannot be predicted with certainty. For example, during the H1N1 pandemic, there was an initial wave of cases in the spring followed by a more severe wave of cases in the early fall in much of the United States. The intervals between pandemics are quite variable and unpredictable, but it is likely that pandemics of influenza will continue to occur in the future.

Taken from the CDC website, the following is an in-depth look at how the CDC measures disease progression.

The Pandemic Intervals Framework (PIF) describes the progression of an influenza pandemic using six intervals. This framework is used to guide influenza pandemic planning and provides recommendations for risk assessment, decision-making, and action in the United States. These intervals provide a common method to describe pandemic activity which can inform public health actions. The duration of each pandemic interval might vary depending on the characteristics of the virus and the public health response.

1) Investigation of cases of novel influenza A virus infection in humans

When novel influenza A viruses are identified in people, public health actions focus on targeted monitoring and investigation. This can trigger a risk assessment of that virus with the Influenza Risk Assessment Tool (IRAT), which is used to evaluate if the virus has the potential to cause a pandemic.

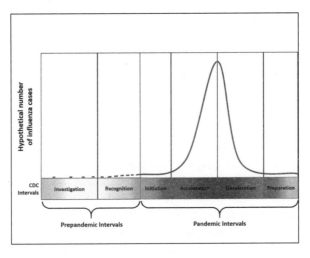

2) Recognition of increased potential for ongoing transmission of a novel influenza A virus

When increasing numbers of human cases of novel influenza A illness are identified and the virus has the potential to spread from person-to-person, public health actions focus on control of the outbreak, including treatment of sick persons.

3) Initiation of a pandemic wave

A pandemic occurs when people are easily infected with a novel influenza A virus that has the ability to spread in a sustained manner from person-to-person.

4) Acceleration of a pandemic wave

The acceleration (or "speeding up") is the upward epidemiological curve as the new virus infects susceptible people. Public health actions at this time may focus on the use of appropriate non-pharmaceutical interventions in the community (e.g. school and child-care facility closures, social distancing), as well the use of medications (e.g. antivirals) and vaccines, if available. These actions combined can reduce the spread of the disease and prevent illness or death.

5) Deceleration of a pandemic wave

The deceleration (or "slowing down") happens when pandemic influenza cases consistently decrease in the United States. Public health actions include continued vaccination, monitoring of pandemic influenza A virus circulation and illness, and reducing the use of non-pharmaceutical interventions in the community (e.g. school closures).

6) Preparation for future pandemic waves

When pandemic influenza has subsided, public health actions include continued monitoring of pandemic influenza A virus activity and preparing for potential additional waves of infection. It is possible that a 2nd pandemic wave could have higher severity than the initial wave. An influenza pandemic is declared ended when enough data shows that the influenza virus, worldwide, is similar to a seasonal influenza virus in how it spreads and the severity of the illness it can cause.

In addition to describing the progression of a pandemic, certain indicators and assessments are used to define when one interval moves into another. CDC uses two tools (the Influenza Risk Assessment Tool and the Pandemic Severity Assessment Framework) to evaluate the pandemic risk that a new influenza A virus can pose. The results from both of these assessments are used to guide federal, state, and local public health decisions.

How the CDC measures the severity of disease and pandemics

Health organizations have steps in place to monitor and measure diseases around the world in order to strategically classify if a disease is a pandemic. The following is an excerpt from the CDC's website identifying the necessary steps they use.

Step 1: Identify and Evaluate Measures of Transmissibility and Severity: We first identified epidemiologic measures that may be indicators of either the transmissibility of a novel influenza virus or the clinical severity in infected persons. The identification of relevant measures within these categories was based on an extensive review of historical seasonal and pandemic influenza literature, including published articles and reports of surveillance data collected from the 1918 pandemic forward. Three criteria were used to evaluate the identified measures: 1) the availability and quality of data related to the measures during the early stages of past influenza pandemics and seasonal influenza epidemics; 2) the presence of enough variation in the measure to produce a biologically plausible and measurable scale; and 3) the epidemiologic strengths and limitations of the measure (Technical Appendix).

Step 2: Scaling Measures of Transmissibility and Severity: From the list of measures identified in step 1, we abstracted data from the literature review on the measures as reported during previous influenza seasons and pandemics. To create a comparable scale across the various measures of transmissibility and clinical severity, we first identified the range of values that had been observed historically for each measure. The data for each measure were then categorized into a uniform scale that was consistent across indicators of transmissibility and across indicators of clinical severity.

Because the availability and quality of epidemiologic information will increase throughout the course of a pandemic, we divided the assessment process into 2 assessment frameworks: 1) an "initial assessment" when data are sparse or very uncertain, and 2) a "refined assessment" when data are more available and more certain. A uniform scale of the transmissibility and clinical severity indicators was developed for each framework. When transmission of a novel influenza virus is identified, early epidemiologic measures provide a broad initial assessment, albeit with a high level of uncertainty, and were categorized by using a broad dichotomous scale. The assessment framework would become more refined as additional epidemiologic and clinical information are gathered and the biases in the earliest measures are better characterized. During this period, a similar general framework would incorporate a finer scale, allowing for more discrete separation of seasonal epidemics and pandemics.

Step 3: Summarize and Score Available Measures: During the initial assessment, a combination of the dichotomous scale for indicators of transmissibility and the dichotomous scale for indicators of severity results in a framework with 4 profiles (A, B, C, D). An initial assessment can be made as soon as data on some measures become available and would continue to be reviewed and revised as the data warrant. As early data become available, issues of data quality are also essential to consider.

Step 4: Provide Historical Context: For the refined assessment, we scaled and plotted data from obtained from our literature review for 4 pandemics (2009, 1968, 1957, 1918) and 3 non-pandemic influenza seasons that ranged in transmissibility and severity (1978–79, 2006–07, and 2007–08) (Technical Appendix). When multiple measures for transmissibility or severity were present, we used the median score across all available measures. Age-stratified data from the 2009 influenza A (H1N1) pandemic were also similarly scaled and plotted by using the age categories <18 years, 18–64 years, and >65 years.

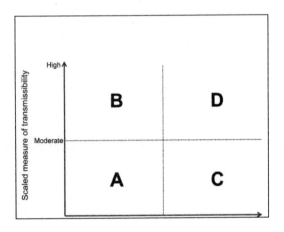

What Makes Coronavirus a Pandemic

Our growing population, vast array of transportation systems, ease in global travel, and all-around accessibility can cause infectious disease to easily spread far more rapidly compared to any other time in recorded history.

Given those factors, with coronavirus threatening multiple countries, this could be a perfect storm for a full-blown pandemic. As coronavirus sweeps the globe, many are wondering why the WHO and CDC have not declared this a pandemic yet.

First and foremost, the CDC and WHO organizations are constantly learning how to better adapt the knowledge they glean from recent epidemics in order to have better response times for future ones. In 2014, the CDC updated their pandemic response framework to reflect the lessons learned from the 2009 H1N1 pandemic and recent responses to outbreaks of novel flu viruses, such as the swine-origin variant H3N2 (H3N2v).

The six phases outlined in the revised plan are:

1. Investigation of cases of novel flu in humans or animals
2. Recognition of increased potential for ongoing trans-mission
3. Initiation of a pandemic wave, meaning efficient and sustained transmission
4. Acceleration of a pandemic wave, meaning a consis-tently increasing number of cases in the United States
5. Deceleration of a pandemic wave, defined as consis-tently declining cases in the United States
6. Preparation for future pandemic waves, meaning low pandemic flu activity

In early March 2020, the CDC stated, "The risk from these outbreaks depends on characteristics of the virus, including how well it spreads between people, the severity of resulting illness, and the medical or other measures available to con-trol the impact of the virus (for example, vaccine or treatment medications). The fact that this disease has caused illness, in-cluding illness resulting in death, and sustained person-to-per-son spread is concerning. These factors meet two of the criteria of a pandemic. As community spread is detected in more and more countries, the world moves closer toward meeting the third criteria—worldwide spread of the new virus." On March 11th, the WHO determined that coronavirus does meet the third criteria for a pandemic: worldwide community spread.

Community Spread: What to Expect with Coronavirus

Before February 27, 2020, the fears surrounding the coro-navirus were regarding those who traveled to the areas of China that were affected by the disease. But that day changed everything. It was announced that the first case of coronavirus from an "unknown origin" had been diagnosed. This suddenly made this biological phenomenon all the more real, thus caus-ing many to open their eyes to the reality that they need to prepare for the long-haul.

"Unknown origin" means the person did not recently travel to a foreign country or have contact with a person known to have the virus. The CDC scrambled to inform the public with this message:

> At this time, the patient's exposure is unknown. It's possible this could be an instance of community spread of COVID-19, which would be the first time this has happened in the United States. Community spread means spread of an illness for which the source of infection is unknown. It's also possible, however, that the patient may have been exposed to a returned traveler who was infected.
>
> This case was detected through the US public health system—picked up by astute clinicians. This brings the total number of COVID-19 cases in the United States to 15.

Within a matter of days four new coronavirus cases spread to communities California, Oregon, and Washington State. The new cases had no travel history or known contact with another case.

With a domestic viral spread, it proved that our biggest fears were here—it was uncontained and out in the open. Simply put, finding sporadic cases of coronavirus in the community was a game changer. Not only for the CDC, who shifted their course of action from containment to a mitigation strategy, but for the citizens who now had to change their response toward action and preparation.

It is unknown if the spread of this virus will be slow or fast moving. What we do know is that local and state governments are preparing for the fact that the spread will continue and cause a dramatic shift in how communities operate, which is already happening. As the government sees fit, they are activating pandemic mitigation measures. For example, pandemic mitigation measures that have occurred during an influenza pandemic include:

- Breakdowns in communications, supply chains, payroll service issues, and healthcare staff shortages should be anticipated when preparing for a pandemic.
- Isolation and treatment (as appropriate) with influenza antiviral medications of all persons with confirmed or probable pandemic influenza. Isolation may occur in the home or healthcare setting, depending on the severity of the individual's illness and/or the current capacity of the healthcare infrastructure.
- Voluntary home quarantine of members of households with confirmed or probable influenza case(s) and consideration of combining this intervention with the prophylactic use of antiviral medications, providing sufficient quantities of effective medications exist and that a feasible means of distributing them is in place.
- Dismissal of students from schools (including public and private schools as well as colleges and universities) and school-based activities and closure of childcare programs, coupled with protecting children and teenagers through social distancing in the community to achieve reductions of out-of-school social contacts and community mixing.
- Use of social distancing measures to reduce contact between adults in the community and workplace, including, for example, cancellation of large public gatherings and alteration of workplace environments and schedules to decrease social density and preserve a healthy workplace to the greatest extent possible without disrupting essential services. Enable institutions of workplace leave policies that align incentives and facilitate adherence with the nonpharmaceutical interventions.

How Will the Federal, State, and Local Governments Respond?

When localized cases begin spreading into multiple states, government response occurs at the federal, state, and local governments. While there are many who criticize the responses, they are in place to ensure cohesion between the government channels and ensures the stability of the country.

A government-centric approach is not enough to meet the challenges posed by a catastrophic incident. Focus has shifted to a "whole community approach," which leverages all of the resources of a community in preparing for, protecting against, responding to, recovering from, and mitigating against all hazards. Here are some excerpts from the *National Strategy for Pandemic Influenza Implementation Plan*:

> The goals of the Federal Government response to a pandemic are to: (1) stop, slow, or otherwise limit the spread of a pandemic to the United States; (2) limit the domestic spread of a pandemic, and mitigate disease, suffering and death; and (3) sustain infrastructure and mitigate impact to the economy and the functioning of society.

While the main goal is, of course, to prevent epidemics from spiraling out of control and infecting larger populations, as we have seen with the public's response to the coronavirus, there are other factors the government must consider: political, economic, socioeconomic.

> The economic and societal disruption of an influenza pandemic could be significant. Absenteeism across multiple sectors related to personal illness, illness in family members, fear of contagion, or public health measures to limit contact with others could threaten the functioning of critical infrastructure, the movement of goods and services, and operation of institutions such as schools and universities. A pandemic

would thus have significant implications for the economy, national security, and the basic functioning of society.[6]

As such, there are laws and executive orders in place to ensure the safety of the public, and that the infrastructure, economy, and national security can continue to function during a pandemic event. The executive orders in place will effectively transfer, even for a limited time, critical industries and business sectors to federal government control. Examples of this are food production facilities, trucking, and train power. In the case of coronavirus or other deadly pathogens, pharmaceutical production and medical equipment production will be prioritized according to the nation's needs.

Some of these laws and executive orders involve what many feel to be extreme measures to control communicable diseases. These laws apply to those who are infected as well as to healthy citizens who have no existing symptoms. Additionally, an executive order signed by President Obama allows for the "apprehension, detention, or conditional release of individuals to prevent the introduction, transmission, or spread of suspected communicable diseases."

It is important to emphasize that we are not left alone to our devices during these critical times. Our federal, state, and local government have emergency preparedness plans in place and, after 9/11, all maintain budgets to deal with crisis scenarios. Ideally, if they have planned appropriately, they will be able to work effectively to, perhaps not prevent a crisis but to respond and mitigate effectively and efficiently. That's not to say you shouldn't prepare your own person and familial preparedness plan.

There are many moving parts when it comes to pandemic preparedness. Coordinating local, state, and federal government entities, as well as ensuring the country's infrastructures are sound, and protecting the public during a crisis, is a lot to manage. The bureaucracy is what slows the action response down, but the plans are in place for a reason. While the break-down of intervening governments is complicated, in and of it-self, this is a general overview of what you can expect from your government.

The federal government:

- Acts to prevent the entry of communicable diseases into the United States. Quarantine and isolation may be used at US ports of entry.
- Is authorized to take measures to prevent the spread of communicable diseases between states.
- May accept state and local assistance in enforcing federal quarantine.
- May assist state and local authorities in preventing the spread of communicable diseases.

State, local, and tribal authorities:

- Enforce isolation and quarantine within their borders.

It is possible for federal, state, local, and tribal health authorities to have and use all at the same time separate but co-existing legal quarantine power in certain events. In the event of a conflict, federal law is supreme.

Censorship of Information

Public information will carefully be crafted in order to avoid panic. This occurred in previous pandemics, and it is occurring now. For instance, because a world war was raging during the Spanish Flu of 1918, countries like Britain, France, Germany, and other European countries wanted to avoid their opponents knowing an illness was being passed through the troops. They made the decision to censor that in the news in order to avoid the other side thinking they had an upper hand. Incidentally, Spain, a neutral country, was the only country to be forthcoming about the flu in its country and reported it in their newspapers. When the second wave of this pandemic hit, because Spain was the one who reported it first, the virus was dubbed "The Spanish Flu."

Many believe information about the Coronavirus is being censored. Calls to remain calm and not to panic have been echoed for weeks from the White House as well in other countries. However, after the first confirmed coronavirus death in Washington state, panic shopping from concerned citizens ensued. The response to stock up on supplies was apocalyptic in nature. In a Costco in Hawaii, employees were limiting shoppers to five packages each of toilet paper and paper towels and hand loading them into carts. As pallet after pallet was cleaned out, many customers had to leave and come back at another time because supplies simply sold out.

As well, another possible censorship is regarding whether or not to wear facemasks. A vast majority of people are erring on the side of caution and rushing out to include N95 and N100 respirators in their preparedness supplies. Officials are indicating this is causing a face mask shortage.

The CDC has admitted that there is a shortage of PPE (personal protective equipment) including face masks for healthcare professionals and encouraged concerned citizens that it is not necessary to wear a mask.

CDC's Recommendations for Using a Facemask

With fears of COVID-19 sweeping the planet, shortages are leaving doctors, nurses, and other frontline workers dangerously ill-equipped to care for COVID-19 on the front lines. This fracture in medical supplies is leaving many in the healthcare industry exposed to possibly contracting this deadly pathogen from infected patients or infecting others because they have been exposed. Moreover, this takes essential nurses off the care lines and into quarantine, opening up another shortage of critical medical staff.

The CDC does not recommend that people who are well wear a facemask to protect themselves from respiratory diseases, including COVID-19. They believe that facemasks should be used by people who show symptoms of COVID-19 to help prevent the spread of the disease to others. The use of face-masks is also crucial for health workers and people who are taking care of someone in close settings (at home or in a health care facility).

Considering that coronaviruses spread from infected water droplets, we can assume a mask that seals to the face would be more effective than no measure taken at all. Using a disposable mask will prevent you from touching your nose and/or mouth, which is how the virus enters the body.

The fact that most of us touch our faces 90 times a day, it would be beneficial to find a way to protect those points of entry. Despite the Surgeon Generals recommendations to not have a facemask, during times of pandemic fear, we advise the opposite. It is both practical and essential to have a protec-tive barrier to filter out infected moist droplets in the air in conjunction with a way to protect the hands from coming in contact with the virus.

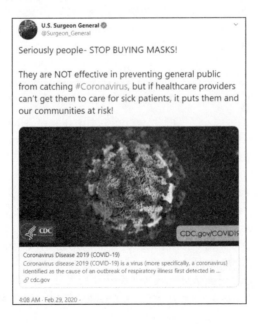

As well, if you are going to a crowded area, plan on being at an airport or flying on an airplane, on a crowded bus or subway, you will be amongst people in tight quarters that could make the usage of a surgical mask, at least, a good one.

FEMA Response Plans

If state or local governments become overwhelmed as a result of an incident or disaster, the president declare a "major disaster" or "emergency" in response and authorizes assistance through other public health emergency response authorities like FEMA.

Utilizing the Robert T. Stafford Disaster Relief and Emergency Assistance Act which is a federal law designed to bring an orderly and systemic means of federal natural disaster assistance for state and local governments in carrying out their responsibilities to aid citizens, FEMA ensures continuity of public assistance during times of a health crisis. Under an emergency declaration, FEMA may provide assistance for emergency protective measures. FEMA provides supplemental assistance for State and local government recovery expenses, and the Federal share will always be at least 75 percent of the eligible costs.

When activated, FEMA responds to emergencies by providing assistance in the following categories:

- Transportation
- Communications
- Public Works and Engineering
- Firefighting
- Information and Planning
- Mass Care, Emergency Assistance, Housing, and Human Services
- Logistics Management and Resource Support
- Public Health and Medical Services
- Search and Rescue
- Oil and Hazardous Materials Response

- Agriculture and Natural Resources
- Energy
- Public Safety and Security
- Long-Term Community Recovery
- External Affairs

When activated, in times of a contagious disease event or pandemic crisis, FEMA will serve a vital function, especially when large communities are under mandatory quarantine. They will be able transport necessary supplies across the country, train necessary health workers on public safety, create emergency medical facilities, create emergency barriers to ensure public safety, and provide emergency communications if utilities stop running.

Enforcement

If a quarantinable disease is suspected or identified, CDC may issue a federal isolation or quarantine order. Public health authorities at the federal, state, local, and tribal levels may sometimes seek help from police or other law enforcement officers to enforce a public health order. US Customs and Border Protection and US Coast Guard officers are authorized to help enforce federal quarantine orders. Breaking a federal quarantine order is punishable by fines and imprisonment. Federal law allows the conditional release of persons from quarantine if they comply with medical monitoring and surveillance.

In the CDC's *Interim Pre-pandemic Planning Guidance: Community Strategy for Pandemic Influenza Mitigation in the United States*, we see the following measures, many of which could also apply to coronavirus:

- Isolation and treatment (as appropriate) with influenza antiviral medications of all persons with confirmed or probable pandemic influenza. Isolation may occur in the home or healthcare setting, depending on the severity of the individual's illness and/or the current capacity of the healthcare infrastructure.

- Voluntary home quarantine of members of households with confirmed or probable influenza case(s) and consideration of combining this intervention with the prophylactic use of antiviral medications, providing sufficient quantities of effective medications exist and that a feasible means of distributing them is in place.

- Dismissal of students from schools (including public and private schools as well as colleges and universities) and school-based activities and closure of childcare programs, coupled with protecting children and teenagers through social distancing in the community to achieve reductions of out-of-school social contacts and community mixing.

- Use of social distancing measures to reduce contact between adults in the community and workplace, including, for example, cancellation of large public gatherings and alteration of workplace environments and schedules to decrease social density and preserve a healthy workplace to the greatest extent possible without disrupting essential services. Enable institutions of workplace leave policies that align incentives and facilitate adherence with the nonpharmaceutical interventions (NPIs) outlined above.

The Division of Global Migration and Quarantine (DGMQ)

To protect and prevent the introduction, transmission, and spread of communicable diseases in the United States in times of epidemic and pandemic concerns, the health organizations have implemented laws and delegated authority to the Division of Global Migration and Quarantine. The mission of the Division of Global Migration and Quarantine (DGMQ)is to reduce morbidity and mortality among immigrants, refugees, travelers, expatriates, and other globally mobile populations, and to prevent the introduction, transmission, and spread of communicable diseases through regulation, science, research, preparedness, and response.

- Protecting public health at US ports of entry by rapidly responding to sick travelers who arrive in the United States, alerting travelers about disease outbreaks, and restricting the importation of animals and products that may carry disease.
- Keeping Americans healthy during travel and while living abroad by reducing illness and injury among US residents traveling internationally or living abroad through alerts, recommendations, education, and support—based on the best science—to travelers and healthcare providers.
- Ensuring the health of individuals coming to live and work in the United States by overseeing the mandatory health screenings for all immigrants and refugees entering the United States, as well as overseas vaccination and parasite treatment programs.
- Partnering to protect the health of US communities along the US-Mexico border by working with state, local, and Mexican public health institutions to detect, notify, investigate, and respond to reports of illness and infectious disease among residents and travelers in US communities along the US-Mexico border.

The Final Rule for Control of Communicable Diseases

The final rule for the Control of Communicable Diseases includes amendments to the current domestic (interstate) and foreign quarantine regulations for the control of communicable diseases.

The Final Rule:

- Outlines the provisions to reflect input received from individuals, industry, state and federal partners, public health authorities, and other interested parties.
- Does not authorize compulsory medical testing, vaccination, or medical treatment without prior informed consent.
- Requires CDC to advise individuals subject to medical examinations that such examinations will be conducted by an authorized health worker and with prior informed consent.
- Includes strong due process protections for individuals subject to public health orders, including a right to counsel for indigent individuals.
- Does not expand CDC's authority beyond what is granted by Congress, nor does it alter the list of diseases subject to federal isolation or quarantine, which is established by an Executive Order of the President.
- Limits to 72 hours the amount of time that an individual may be apprehended pending the issuance of a federal order for isolation, quarantine, or conditional release.
- Provides the public with explicit information about how and where the CDC conducts public health risk assessments and manages travelers at US ports of entry.

Societal Impact

Perhaps the most ominous of all is the concern for supply disruptions. Providers already face a global disruption in medical supplies and the more this virus continues to wage on in the United States, the more stressed the country's supply chain will become.

The difficulty that government officials have with managing widespread pandemics is balancing the need for rapid medical response with other critical aspects of our society that could have a devastating impact on life as we know it.

Everything from healthcare and insurance to food supply chains and retirement accounts come into play when we start discussing worst-case mitigation strategies for widespread pandemic scenarios.

The problem we face is that taking action, even when justified, could lead to immediate shocks to parts of our lives that we often take for granted.

The threat to global supply chains and just in time delivery

As China began locking down entire regions in response to the rapid and deadly spread of this novel virus, it became apparent very quickly that the majority of the manufacturing base for the United States had essentially come to a standstill. One estimate indicated that as many as 74% of all Chinese factory workers were forced to stay home.

In addition to the low cost garments and electronics, we source a lot of raw materials and essential products from China including the base elements for the production of life-saving pharmaceutical drugs, meats like chicken and beef, and yes, even the N95 masks that are at the time of this writing selling for 25 times their normal going price.

The FDA admits that concerns of a global COVID-19 outbreak would likely impact the medical product supply chain, including potential disruptions to supply or shortages of critical medical products in the US.

In a report, they state, "the FDA has been closely monitoring the supply chain with the expectation that the COVID-19 outbreak would likely impact the medical product supply chain, including potential disruptions to supply or shortages of critical medical products in the U.S."

Overall, this remains an evolving and very dynamic issue. We are committed to continuing to communicate with the public as we have further updates.

We also continue to aggressively monitor the market for any firms marketing products with fraudulent COVID-19 diagnosis, prevention or treatment claims. The FDA can and will use every authority at our disposal to protect consumers from bad actors who take advantage of a crisis to deceive the public, including pursuing warning letters, seizures or injunctions against products on the market that are not in compliance with the law, or against firms or individuals who violate the law.

The agency reached out to 63 companies with a total of 72 facilities in China that make essential medical devices and at this time, no shortages have been reported. But that may be short-lived and as we keep hearing in this ordeal, "it may not be a question of if, but when."

In fact, World Health Organization Director-General Tedros Adhanom Ghebreyesus told reporters "the world is facing severe disruption in the market for personal protective equipment." At the time, he reported backlogs of four to six months, demand that was up to 100 times greater than usual and prices up to 20 times higher. Personal Protective Equipment or PPE may include items such as gloves, eye protection, full protective body suits, and N95 respirators.

In and of itself, that's a problem we can deal with if it is short term, and China is already making moves to ensure they have at least some factories that are operational, as they understand the threat that shutting down businesses poses to their multi-trillion dollar manufacturing economy.

Here in the United States, supply lines being cut off has a different, but equally as detrimental, impact to society.

What we've seen in the United States in the weeks following the news is runs on grocery stores and bulk suppliers. While initially isolated to cities in and around areas where contagion has appeared, eventually the panic spreads.

As officials in local areas begin declaring emergencies, suggesting home quarantines and shutting down schools, conferences, and other venues where large groups gather, people will realize that their pantries are empty and they need to stock up on a couple of week's worth of food. They will head to their local grocery store and see that the lines out the door mean there will be nothing left once they get inside. So, they'll head to a nearby suburban store or out to a rural area in search of goods.

As this flow of individuals from major cities spiders out to surrounding areas, it will cause local residents to rush to grocery stores to ensure they get their own emergency supplies.

In modern times, the United States has been able to mitigate such supply crunches during heightened states of emergency by sourcing supplies from other regions and delivering them quickly to impacted areas.

But what happens when there is a run on supplies everywhere and all at once?

The best we can hope for in such a scenario is that retailers have some stores in their warehouses and that they'll deliver those goods just in time for you to need them, just like they always do. But this is more than likely wishful thinking.

From a preparedness standpoint, you have to assume that once the store shelves are cleared out, they won't be resupplied for weeks.

To prepare for supply line disruptions, your approach should be, "if I don't have it, I am not going to get it."

One could argue that the government has been stockpiling supplies for years. In fact, billions of dollars have been spent to stockpile pandemic masks, emergency blankets, beds, emergency meals, medicines, and scores of other critical supplies for the US population, but when we consider that there are 300 million Americans, we must assume that even 100 million reserve emergency meals will not be enough to support the entire population.

These disruptions to the supply chain pose a serious risk at every level of society. Healthcare workers may not have access to protective equipment, critically ill patients may have no access to critical medicines, and families will not be able to restock their kitchens.

The stress will lead to desperation, which could lead to a cascading breakdown in other parts of our society.

Assuming more and more people stay home in self-quarantine, other services within our economy could be in trouble. For example, if electrical workers, water plant workers, phone network technicians, and delivery truck drivers have to stay home, then the proper functioning of utilities, supplies of gas, and internet delivery of goods could be disrupted.

Could There be a Run on Financial Markets?

Should pandemic mitigation strategies employed by first responders and government officials go to the same extremes as what we've seen in other countries, we need to consider the potential impact on our economy, as well as financial markets.

We're all invested in the US economy in one way or another, and as quarantines become commonplace, we can assume that swaths of people will stay home from school and work. A large number of Americans don't get paid when they don't work, which means that when next month's bills come due, they won't have the money to cover their rent or mortgage, utilities, credit card payments, car payments, or student loans.

The financial breakdown will start on the individual level and very quickly progress to banks and creditors.

In short, if we experience a home quarantine period nationwide for several weeks to months, a lot of people aren't going to be able to pay their bills, and that includes major corporations (who can no longer sell products, or even get them because their parts supplier is in China).

As news of the seriousness of the pandemic breaks, financial markets around the global go into freefall.

Not everyone is invested in stock and bond markets, but nonetheless, a lot of people are, including retirees who depend on a monthly stipend from their investment. We're talking about millions of people who could see their life savings cut in half in just a matter of weeks as panic selling takes hold.

If you've ever witnessed what happens during financial crashes, the short version is: everyone sells in the hopes of maintaining at least some savings.

While the government will attempt to infuse markets with lower interest rates and perhaps even cash subsidies directly to individuals financially affected by crisis, the collapse of markets could be so overwhelming on a global scale that it could take months to stabilize and years to regain value.

A Breakdown of Law and Order

For some, especially those who did not prepare reserve supplies in time, desperate times may lead to desperate measures.

We've already seen and read the reports from around the world that frontline medical workers and law enforcement personnel can get infected just like the rest of us.

Assuming a similar infection rate to the general population, we can expect many frontline personnel to be unavailable to respond to emergency calls, which means that the criminal element in our society will run rampant. They'll start with looking for high dollar goods, as usual, and will also be looking for resources like food and medicine. When they don't find what they need at your local shops, they will begin targeting apartments and homes, posing a serious risk to safety.

Should local law enforcement be overwhelmed, it is possible, and very much part of our national emergency plan, to activate emergency policing and enforcement on a State or Federal level. Such measures will likely be taken as needed, city-by-city, and may be fairly effective. But such a response has never been attempted on a national level to respond to a widespread crisis.

Thus, from a security standpoint, one must assume no help is coming, so considering home security procedures and preparations is a must.

Travel Lockdown

We've already seen the United States implement travel restrictions from pandemic hot zones. But such restrictions were too late, as potentially thousands of infected individuals travelled on airlines, trains, and with ride shares.

Should the government begin self-quarantine restrictions, we can expect that such a move will come with widespread travel restrictions, as well. And we're not just talking about international travel.

To successfully stop the spread of any contagion with a high rate of infection, officials will need to stop the movement of the population. Thus, we can assume that air travel, bus travel, train travel, and all ride share services could be suspended on a nationwide level, stranding us at home for potentially weeks and months.

Were our officials to follow measures similar to what China enacted, a travel lockdown would mean that you wouldn't be able to travel from city to city, or even take a trip outside your home more than once per week to get essential supplies from emergency distribution sites.

While such a strategy would be drastic and was unemployable at the onset of a pandemic due to lack of information about the dangers of a novel virus, once the danger is confirmed it is the only way to slow the spread of a deadly pandemic in order to buy time for researchers to manufacture treatment options or vaccines.

An Overwhelmed Healthcare System

In a warning to Americans, Liz Specht, PhD, estimates that there are about 2.8 hospital beds per 1,000 people in the United States. That's roughly one million total beds. As Dr. Specht notes, "at any given time, 65% of those beds are already occupied. That leaves about 330,000 beds available nationwide."

Specht goes on to explain that should just 1% of the 300 million Americans catch a virus like COVID19, which has a hospitalization rate of about 10%, all beds in America would be taken.

And while FEMA has preparedness plans to deploy mobile hospitals by utilizing military transport to move around the country, some researchers have suggested that tens of millions of Americans could be infected in a short time frame, potentially requiring millions of hospital beds that we simply do not have available.

Even if we did have enough beds available, the other problem we face is what some have referred to as a "run on the hospitals," which would overwhelm even non-emergency healthcare services as tens of millions of Americans concerned with infection race to local clinics and hospitals seeking help.

Consider how long you have to sit in the waiting room when you have an appointment. Now consider what that wait will look like when there are 50 people in line in front of you when you arrive.

The massive influx of sick people needing to be seen by a doctor could run into another problem even if they get face-to-face time with a medical practitioner. There may be no treatment options available! As of this writing, viral researchers are exploring the use of anti-viral medicines and are working on a vaccine, but there may simply not be enough existing anti-viral medications, oxygen ventilators, or IV fluid bags for everyone who needs them due to overwhelming demand coupled with the supply crunch on raw materials.

Medical Bills and Deductibles Could Be Massive

As of this writing, Governor Newsom of California has ordered health insurance providers in the State to offer all COVID-19 testing free of charge. With large medical insurance deductibles looming for millions of Americans who may be staying home from work and not being paid their regular salary, medical bills could prove to be a double whammy for an already cash-strapped American public.

It has been reported that a standard test for Coronavirus could cost as much as $3500, though costs are estimated to drop.

Nonetheless, testing for a family of four could easily cost $10,000, and that's before other expenses like emergency room care, or in a worst case, hospitalization that could easily run into the tens of thousands for those with a serious infection requiring potentially weeks of care (if it's even available). As of 3/11/2020, in a statement to the nation regarding the rapidly unfolding situation with COVID-19, Trump stated that major health insurers would not only cover the costs of coronavirus treatment in insurance plans, but also waive co-payments for all coronavirus treatments.

On an individual level, these bills would be significantly more than most Americans can pay, the effective of which could be disastrous to health insurance companies and healthcare providers.

It should be noted that anyone who seeks treatment will receive it if possible and will not be rejected due to financial issues. So in that respect, all Americans do have emergency healthcare available to them should they need it. Paying for it, however, is a whole other matter and one that could lead to the collapse of major insurance carriers or hospital networks.

While it's not being publicized, Federal and State governments are working on solutions to this aspect of the problem and it will more than likely come in the form of emergency bailouts similar to what was done with banks following the financial crash of 2008.

Electricity, Water, Sewage, Sanitation, and Internet Failures

In a widespread pandemic scenario we have to assume that if we and our families are staying in home quarantine, so, too, are all of the millions of people who maintain our nation's infrastructure. This means that all those people involved in making sure your lights turn on, your water is clean, your toilet flushes, and that you can still access your favorite online portals aren't going to be there when our basic services require emergency maintenance.

As certain services break down, even more panic could set in.

Electricity

During the California power outages in 2019, generators across the state sold out as the primary electricity provider engaged in widespread power shutdowns affecting millions of residents. And while those outages lasted just a few days at a time, it gave the general public a peek into what a long-term outage lasting weeks could look like.

Those with electric stoves, heaters, and air conditioners were, at worst, inconvenienced for a few days. For some, however, power outages were life threatening. Those requiring refrigeration of their medicine or electricity to run ventilators could have died had there not been immediate healthcare services available. Many hospitals maintain generators to provide essential care during an outage, but as noted previously, what happens if the healthcare system is overwhelmed or generator gas supply lines are disrupted and those requiring electrically powered equipment can't get it to turn on?

Water

Without water for three days, humans will die, which is why this preparedness aspect is so critical for emergencies. We saw in the aftermath of Hurricane Katrina what happens when clean water filtration is out of service. It took emergency responders nearly five days to get water to the Super Dome, a blaring warning sign of just how susceptible we are to disruptions and how bureaucracy during crisis could lead to preventable deaths.

Our emergency responders knew the hurricane was coming and it still overwhelmed us. Now imagine a water plant crisis that we didn't see coming in just two major cities simultaneously, during a pandemic when there isn't enough staff to respond, and all water supplies in the region have been stripped.

It's easy to see how this could pose a significant problem.

Sanitation and Sewage

Another major but often overlooked factor during crisis is sanitation and sewage. We've seen time and again that disease spreads rapidly following an emergency event when sanitation services crumble. It has been reported that following the 2010 earthquake in Haiti, more people died from disease after the primary earthquake than during the earthquake itself.

Should we find ourselves in a situation requiring a full quarantine, those folks who usually pick up your trash every week aren't going to show up. And it could be weeks before they do. That means trash will build up, leave a horrible smell around your house or apartment, and will likely be ravaged by wild animals and torn open all over your driveway. Spoiled food in and around your immediate area could pose a health hazard.

Our sewage systems could also fail, as there may not be anyone to maintain the plants. This means you won't have anywhere to flush your waste. And while you may be able to use plastic bags to store the waste, should sanitation services not be available at the same time, human waste could be everywhere.

Internet

While at first glance we may think that an internet outage is no big deal because we could just sit down to a good book and maybe hang out in the back yard or on the patio until it comes back on, the fact of the matter is that the internet is an absolutely essential infrastructure component. It's used for, among other things, routing and delivery of goods across the country, financial markets, consumer purchasing, news, and peer-to-peer communication.

Internet outages happen on a daily basis, so they are to be expected. But usually our services are back up and running within a couple of hours. During a pandemic, workers may be too sick to work or quarantined at home, which means outage repair times could be days, perhaps even weeks.

Moreover, non-accidental outages involving cyberattacks become much more likely, as nefarious actors and even foreign governments could use the pandemic as an opportunity to infiltrate critical networks.

You already know that you'll probably lose access to social media, email, your favorite websites, and your general flow of information, but internet outages could affect the vast majority of communication services including direct calling and texting to family, friends, and emergency services.

Whether you are on a wireless network or a hardline broadband connection, many networks in a particular local area will have just a couple of points of failure, so if one type of service goes down, so too does the other.

Likewise, while many of us still have landlines in our homes in addition to our cell phones, just about all of these landlines eventually connect to and transmit our calls utilizing the same underlying internet.

Though such a scenario is unlikely, the ramifications would lead to misinformation, confusion, and panic.

Some local TV and radio stations may still operate, providing an important medium for information during an internet outage.

It Can Happen All At Once

We regularly experience disruptions to important sectors of our economy and infrastructure without much fanfare. The public sector and private companies have personnel and procedures to deal with failures. Usually these failures are mere inconveniences.

In a pandemic scenario, however, a lot of things could potentially go wrong simultaneously.

There is a systemic risk of cascading breakdowns—it's just how our system is designed. If one critical area experiences crisis and a solution is not rapidly forthcoming, it could easily lead to other systems coming under stress.

We've already seen it with the recent pandemic.

First, China quarantined their citizens, which lead to a shutdown of factory operations throughout the country. This news reached the United States and Europe and people immediately began buying up N95 masks, toilet paper, and other supplies. People started cancelling travel plans and directed disposable income to emergency related products and services.

The potential manufacturing disruptions and lowered sales expectations coupled with travel cancellations and restrictions culminated in a sell-off of stock markets worldwide.

From there, because no verifiable treatment options yet exist, the situation can continue to snowball.

It starts slowly, then it comes all at once.

In the case of Coronavirus, the extent of the first wave of the virus is still unclear. Officials around the world are taking steps to test, treat, and isolate the virus as much as possible. And they may be successful initially.

But the second wave could be even more disruptive and devastating, as the pillars upon which our fragile societies are built break under overwhelming stress.

CHAPTER 3

Quarantine and Isolation

When there is a concern for dangerous communicable diseases spreading, the CDC activates pandemic mitigation measures. Among these measures are isolation and quarantines. These are the first steps in protecting the public by preventing exposure to infected persons or to persons who may be infected.

Isolation and quarantine help protect the public by preventing exposure to people who have or may have a contagious disease. This also provides a person time for the illness to incubate and for the body to start showing signs of illness.

When ethically justified, these measures are implemented to contain and prevent the transmission of an infectious disease and to restore public health. It will last enough time for medical personnel to assess the situation or for the duration of the contagious period.

As well, quarantine and isolations in times of outbreaks assist in protecting human and national security. Human security is to be understood as "safety from constant threats of hunger, disease, crime, and repression."

What to Expect During a Quarantine

Quarantine means separating a person or group of people who have been exposed to a contagious disease but have not developed illness (symptoms) from others who have not been exposed, in order to prevent the possible spread of that disease.

Typically, if someone is under quarantine, it is a voluntary, short-term home confinement where a person is asked to avoid contact with other people and to remain at home until they are no longer contagious. Other measures to control the spread of disease may include restrictions on the assembly of groups of people (for example, school events), cancellation of public events, suspension of public gatherings, and closings of public places (such as theaters and churches).

Quarantine is usually established for the incubation period of the communicable disease, which is the span of time during which people have developed illness after exposure. Generally speaking, the CDC advises people who believe they have been exposed to a contagious disease but not symptomatic to quarantine themselves (i.e. stay at home), monitor themselves for symptoms, and seek medical evaluation if symptoms appear.

Family Quarantine at Home

Sometimes loved ones become ill and the family must quarantine themselves as a result. Being under quarantine is very unique in that you will not be able to run to the store if your food supplies run out. You must stay confined. Therefore, you need to have everything in place before mitigation measures are activated.

Follow these tips when caring for a sick family member under quarantine:

Only one adult should look after the sick person. It is best if the care person is not pregnant because, depending on the contagious disease, a pregnant woman is at increased risk of complications from many infections.

- Create a sick room (information in Medical Preparedness chapter of this book)
- Use a facemask in quarantine: If you plan on wearing a facemask during quarantine, wear a fitted N95 facemask when helping the sick person. Ensure a good seal has been achieved by sealing the mask over the bridge

of the nose and mouth, and there should be no gaps between the mask and face. Throw away disposable facemasks after one use.

- The sick person should stay in their room, but if they venture out of their room, make sure the sick person wears a facemask.
- Before touching anything else, wash your hands thoroughly with soap and water immediately after taking off a facemask and/or gloves.

Sensory deprivation

Everyone reacts differently to stressful situations such as an infectious disease outbreak that requires social distancing, quarantine, or isolation. If you are unfortunately exposed to a contagious disease and are quarantined, prepare yourself for the possibility of being in complete home isolation for weeks or maybe even months, in some cases, depending on the epidemic or pandemic. Because we are all different, we may have different reactions:

People may feel:

- Anxiety, worry, or fear related to your own health status or the health status of others whom you may have exposed to the disease
- Concern about the resentment that your friends and family may feel if they need to go into quarantine as a result of contact with you
- Discomfort due to the experience of monitoring yourself, or being monitored by others for signs and symptoms of the disease
- Worry regarding time taken off from work and the potential loss of income and job security
- Stress regarding the challenges of securing things you need, such as groceries and personal care items

- Concern about being able to effectively care for children or others in your care
- Uncertainty or frustration about how long you will need to remain in this situation
- Uncertainty about the future
- Loneliness associated with feeling cut off from the world and from loved ones
- Anger if you think you were exposed to the disease because of others' negligence
- Boredom and frustration because you may not be able to work or engage in regular day-to-day activities
- Uncertainty or ambivalence about the situation
- A desire to use alcohol or drugs to cope
- Symptoms of depression, such as feelings of hopelessness, changes in appetite, or sleeping too little or too much
- Symptoms of post-traumatic stress disorder (PTSD), such as intrusive distressing memories, flashbacks (reliving the event), nightmares, changes in thoughts and mood, and being easily startled

We are social creatures, so it makes sense that being in isolation, unable to go out in the world, would have a negative effect on someone. Incidentally, these mental health effects are in direct correlation to the length of time you are in quarantine. If you or a loved one experience any of these reactions for 2 to 4 weeks or more, contact your health care provider.

Reducing boredom while in quarantine at home

It does not matter what age you are, being confined to home for an extended period of time can cause boredom, stress, and conflict. If you have time ahead of the quarantine, these suggestions may help keep the boredom away.

- Arrange with your boss to work from home, if possible.

- Ask your child's school to supply assignments, work sheets, and homework by post or email.
- Take everyone's needs into account as much as possible when you plan activities. Remember, you don't have to spend every moment of quarantine together. Make sure everyone gets the opportunity to spend some time alone.
- Don't rely too heavily on the television and technology. Treat quarantine as an opportunity to do some of those things you never usually have time for, such as board games, crafts, drawing, and reading.
- Accept that conflict and arguments may occur. Try to resolve issues quickly. Distraction may work with young children.

50 Things to Do During Home Quarantine

Here are 50 things to do after you have napped and watched movie marathons.

1. Organize your preparedness supplies
2. Set up your isolation or sick room
3. Start a hobby (learn to knit, make survival bracelets, draw, paint, etc.)
4. Take a few online courses or get an online certification. Some are even free!
5. Read The Prepper's Blueprint or the other books you haven't had a chance to read
6. Make some natural household cleaners
7. Organize the house
8. Finally, get around to the honey-do list and fix things around the house
9. Make some freezer meals
10. Write a book
11. Watch documentaries or movies
12. Start a daily journal
13. Document your struggle against boredom and take a

picture every hour
14. Rearrange your house
15. Practice yoga
16. Exercise
17. Meditate or pray
18. Talk to friends and family
19. Learn how to play an instrument
20. Play a joke on other family members and swap their closet contents with yours
21. Make homemade yogurt
22. Cut your hair
23. Make a trash can a basketball hoop and throw crumpled up paper for baskets
24. Make a bucket list
25. Plan your next season garden
26. Create your own language and then write a dictionary
27. Play board games, Legos or cards
28. Make crafts out of wine corks
29. Film yourself cooking and talk like Julia Child
30. Relearn the art of the handstand
31. Make homemade cards and write a note to family member and friends
32. Organize old pictures or make a scrapbook
33. Have spa day
34. Make a battery out of pennies
35. Practice martial arts
36. Play hide and seek
37. Master dance moves
38. Upcycle mason jars into home decor
39. Memorize your favorite quote or poem
40. Plan your next trip or vacation
41. Start a Pinterest account
42. Learn about photography and take photos
43. Start a blog
44. Make survival preps out of unused household items
45. Learn the Cups song from Pitch Perfect

46. Learn how to play chess
47. Karaoke like a rock star
48. Have a Nerf gun battle
49. Take a nap
50. Make a list of things to do after you are not quarantined

What to Expect During Isolation at a Medical Facility

There are times when medical professionals feel that hospital-specific isolation is the best care for a patient.

When a patient is suspected of having a contagious disease, the medical professional screening the patient will need to take immediate precautions and wear protective gear such as eye protection, gloves, and a facemask.

In the case of medical professionals screening a potential contagious patient, exceptional care is taken to ensure other hospital patients are not exposed. During the screening process, medical professionals will wear the following personal protective equipment (PPE): goggles, disposable full facemask, pair of disposable nonsterile gloves, NIOSH N95, gown.

The following is an excerpt from the CDC on their protocols for minimizing exposure to virulent diseases such as with COVID-19:

- **Before Arrival**
    - When scheduling appointments, instruct patients and persons who accompany them to call ahead or inform HCP upon arrival if they have symptoms of any respiratory infection (e.g., cough, runny nose, fever) and to take appropriate preventive actions (e.g., wear a facemask upon entry to contain cough, follow triage procedures).
    - If a patient is arriving via transport by emergency medical services (EMS), the driver should contact the receiving emergency department (ED) or

healthcare facility and follow previously agreed upon local or regional transport protocols. This will allow the healthcare facility to prepare for receipt of the patient.

- **Upon Arrival and During the Visit**
  - Take steps to ensure all persons with symptoms of suspected COVID-19 or other respiratory infection (e.g., fever, cough) adhere to respiratory hygiene and cough etiquette, hand hygiene, and triage procedures throughout the duration of the visit. Consider posting visual alerts (e.g., signs, posters) at the entrance and in strategic places (e.g., waiting areas, elevators, cafeterias) to provide patients and HCP with instructions (in appropriate languages) about hand hygiene, respiratory hygiene, and cough etiquette. Instructions should include how to use facemasks or tissues to cover nose and mouth when coughing or sneezing, to dispose of tissues and contaminated items in waste receptacles, and how and when to perform hand hygiene.
  - Ensure that patients with symptoms of suspected COVID-19 or other respiratory infection (e.g., fever, cough) are not allowed to wait among other patients seeking care. Identify a separate, well-ventilated space that allows waiting patients to be separated by 6 or more feet, with easy access to respiratory hygiene supplies. In some settings, medically-stable patients might opt to wait in a personal vehicle or outside the healthcare facility where they can be contacted by mobile phone when it is their turn to be evaluated.
  - Ensure rapid triage and isolation of patients with symptoms of suspected COVID-19 or other respiratory infection (e.g., fever, cough):

- Identify patients at risk for having COVID-19 infection before or immediately upon arrival to the healthcare facility.
- Implement triage procedures to detect persons under investigation (PUI) for COVID-19 during or before patient triage or registration (e.g., at the time of patient check-in) and ensure that all patients are asked about the presence of symptoms of a respiratory infection and history of travel to areas experiencing transmission of SARS-CoV-2, the virus that causes COVID-19, or contact with possible COVID-19 patients.
- Implement respiratory hygiene and cough etiquette (i.e., placing a facemask over the patient's nose and mouth if that has not already been done) and isolate the PUI for COVID-19 in an Airborne Infection Isolation Room (AIIR), if available. See recommendations for "Patient Placement" below.
- Inform infection prevention and control services, local and state public health authorities, and other healthcare facility staff as appropriate about the presence of a person under investigation for COVID-19.
- Provide supplies for respiratory hygiene and cough etiquette, including 60%-95% alcohol-based hand sanitizer (ABHS), tissues, no touch receptacles for disposal, and facemasks at healthcare facility entrances, waiting rooms, patient check-ins, etc.

What happens if someone tests positive for a highly contagious disease?

- The patient suspected (i.e., PUI) will be placed in an AIIR that has been constructed and maintained in accordance with current guidelines.
- If the patient does not require hospitalization they can be discharged to home (in consultation with state or

local public health authorities) if deemed medically and socially appropriate. Pending transfer or discharge, place a facemask on the patient and isolate him/her in an examination room with the door closed. Ideally, the patient should not be placed in any room where room exhaust is recirculated within the building without HEPA filtration.

What is AIIR?

Airborne Infection Isolation Rooms (AIIRs) are equipped with separate ventilation systems to ensure the contagious disease is contained. According to CDC, in order to contain the virus and prevent further infection, patients with known or suspected COVID-19 (i.e., PUI) should be placed in an AIIR that has been constructed and maintained in accordance with current guidelines.

These isolation rooms are designed to isolate a patient who is suspected of, or has been diagnosed with, an airborne infectious disease. The negative-pressure isolation room therefore is designed to help prevent the spread of a disease from an infected patient to others in the hospital.

AIIRs are single patient rooms at negative pressure relative to the surrounding areas, and with a minimum of 6 air changes per hour (12 air changes per hour are recommended for new construction or renovation). Air from these rooms should be exhausted directly to the outside or be filtered through a high-efficiency particulate air (HEPA) filter before recirculation. Room doors should be kept closed except when entering or leaving the room, and entry and exit should be minimized. Facilities should monitor and document the proper negative-pressure function of these rooms.

Current CDC guidance for when it is OK to release someone from isolation is made on a case by case basis and includes meeting all of the following requirements:

7. The patient is free from fever without the use of fever-reducing medications.
8. The patient is no longer showing symptoms, including cough.
9. The patient has tested negative on at least two consecutive respiratory specimens collected at least 24 hours apart.
10. Someone who has been released from isolation is not considered to pose a risk of infection to others.

Effects of Isolation on the Psyche

You may experience mixed emotions, including a sense of relief. If you were isolated because you had the illness, you may feel sadness or anger because friends and loved ones may have unfounded fears of contracting the disease from contact with you, even though you have been determined not to be contagious. The best way to end this common fear is to learn about the disease and the actual risk to others. Moreover, you may be frustrated because you are missing out on working and may be paycheck to paycheck or frustrated because you are losing valuable time in preparing your home and family for a possible outbreak.

Sharing this information and talking to loved ones will often calm fears in others and allow you to reconnect with them. If you or your loved one experiences symptoms of extreme stress—such as trouble sleeping, problems with eating too much or too little, inability to carry out routine daily activities, or using drugs or alcohol to cope—speak to a health care provider.

Training the mind to overcome

When playing stories out in your head, your mind does not know if the story is real or not real, it just plays the story out as it unfolds. If you imagine yourself being decisive, controlling your fears, and behaving rationally, then the mind will only know to act this way in the future. If you imagine yourself hiding, terrified and meek, then you will train your mind to act in this manner.

Maneuvering through a worst-case scenario takes mental preparation, and working through emotions we would rather not deal with. Ultimately, one of the emotions you must conquer is fear. Fear and negative thinking can quickly spread like a virus infecting yourself and others around you. Having overwhelming fear can take you to a fight or flight status and literally cause the brain to be paralyzed into inactivity. One way to circumvent this is through visualization.

Visualization techniques are effective exercises that one can do to safely put themselves in a dangerous situation in order to desensitize oneself to the stress of the situation. In turn, you break through the fears and anxieties of the situation and begin finding plausible ways of dealing with it. These mental "dress rehearsals" are similar to what athletes use to give them a greater edge in performance and countless research studies back this up. In fact, as far as athletic performances go, using visualization exercises improves performance by 45%! Why not use this time-tested tool in mentally preparing for emergencies?

By repeatedly facing threatening situations under calm, controlled emotional conditions, we learn to respond in desired ways, free of threat. A good example would be someone who is paralyzed with germ-related phobias, washing hands, showering, and changing clothes dozens of times daily. By encouraging that person to rehearse cognitive reframing and relaxation methods while gradually exposing themselves to sources of germs, a therapist helps build a sense of safety and mastery. Step by step, the work proceeds to tackle greater challenges, from looking at germ-laden objects in the toilet to quickly touching doorknobs to shaking people's hands and beyond. Quite literally, desensitization reprograms our emotional responses by rewiring our brains.

Staying positive with controlled and purposed action

If you find yourself in quarantine or isolation, the stress, fear, and enormity of this situation can be overwhelming. How do you not go crazy in quarantine or isolation?

It is important to train and learn to control your mind to act in times of difficulty. Admittedly, this is easier said than doen. But breaking things into smaller, more achievable goals makes the overall goal itself easier. These small victories are purposed actions that keep your mind moving in a positive stream. In a dire situation, where multiple people are affected, having these small victories keeps the morale of the group up so that everyone is working toward a common goal: surviving the event.

A key strategy for training the mind to have the right attitude is through mental repetition. Repeating positive reinforcing statements such as, "I will get through this," "Things will get better," or "When I get through this, I'm going to start training for a marathon" trains your mind and prevents it from wanting to give up. This creates resiliency. As well, always keep in mind, whatever the circumstance, that nothing is impossible. All you need is a strategy, problem-solving skills, control over your emotions, a little patience, and practice.

When to Go into a Full-On Lockdown

After an explosion of coronavirus cases that rocked Italy, the country made the decision to quickly lockdown its borders. The mandatory lockdown, which started on Feb. 23, 2020 affected 10 towns in Lombardy and one in Veneto. In March, the whole country was placed in quarantine. To date (as of March 12, 2020), more than 9,000 Italians have contracted the virus, but the Italian government fear more is to come. Trucks can get in and out with bare essentials, but police roadblocks keep everyone else in.

When outbreaks spiral out of control, healthcare officials will suggest social distancing measures in order to contain the outbreak. When this happens, individuals will wonder what steps they need to take to prevent infection. Some of the key questions facing concerned citizens revolve around the concepts of self-quarantine and social distancing.

When do you make the call to bug in or bug out? When is the time to take children out of school? Or to stop going to work? When should you make the decision to go into full pandemic lockdown mode?

If you see these 6 key warnings, it's time to activate your pandemic lockdown plan

When outbreak cases continue to climb, or if the contagion comes close to your community, the time to make preparations for a worst-case scenario is immediate. The following are six key warning signs you should be looking for. When these events come to pass or you see these signals, you should strongly consider implementing a self-quarantine lockdown:

1. Emergency officials say they have the situation under control, but more cases continue to appear in your immediate area.
2. Local and state governments officially declare an emergency.
3. Cases have been identified at your local hospital or at schools in your general vicinity.
4. The general public begins to panic and store shelves start running out of key supplies like food and bottled water.
5. Looting and lawlessness occur within the local community.
6. The virus breaches a 50-mile radius surrounding your home or town.

If these signs begin to appear around you, it's time to seriously consider distancing yourself from society, and especially highly dense venues like retail stores, sporting events, or schools.

If the government won't close their borders, you should close yours

Because each of our circumstances is different and we live in varying population densities, each of us will have to make the best choice based on our specific needs. Some people commute to work, some work from home, and some live in the country where the threat of contagious viruses spreading in high volume is not as much of a concern as urban areas.

Activating social distancing protocols is the best way to avoid contagious diseases altogether. If you are prepared to live in your home for a month or longer without venturing into public areas, then you stand a better chance of surviving a pandemic. If you are able to work from home and live full-time at your bug out retreat, take any remaining supplies you have and go now before the pandemic escalates.

- If you have 6 months' worth of savings, perhaps it is worthwhile to take a leave of absence from your employment and live at your bug out retreat full time until the crisis passes.
- If you do not have the flexibility of working from home and must work in an office or warehouse setting, discuss contingency plans with your employer. In addition to educating employees, companies should review their emergency preparedness plans on how to respond if an employee falls sick on the job. The plan should include communicating with other employees, setting up an isolation room, transporting ill employees to the appropriate medical authorities, protecting employees who come into contact with those who are ill, setting up a disinfecting program, and monitoring contact tracing. Organizations could also consider screening employees at the worksite.

It is paramount that the health system keeps the population safe from the spread of a contagious disease. Protocols and mitigation strategies for quarantining and isolating those that are infected will help contain further spread of this deadly disease.

Social Distancing

Social distancing measures that reduce opportunities for person-to-person virus transmission can help delay the spread and slow the exponential growth of a pandemic. The optimal strategy is to implement these measures simultaneously in places where persons gather.

- School closures and dismissals
- Mass gatherings modifications postponements/cancellations
- Other social distancing measures (e.g., offering telecommuting in workplace or seating students further apart in classrooms)

CHAPTER 4

Pandemic Medical Needs

Catastrophic health events like pandemics have the potential to quickly exhaust resources available for proper response.

According to a study, when pandemics cause large morbidity and mortality spikes, they are much more likely to overwhelm health systems. Overwhelmed health systems and other indirect effects may contribute to a 2.3-fold increase in all-cause mortality during pandemics, although attribution of the causative agent is difficult.

As well, healthcare workers' ability to provide care may be reduced. At the peak of a severe influenza pandemic, up to 40 percent of health care workers might be unable to report for duty because they are ill themselves, need to care for ill family members, need to care for children because of school closures, or are afraid.

With the coronavirus outbreaks taking hold of Europe, Asia, and parts of the US, cases continue to increase in multiple countries, and doctors and medical experts are still at a loss re regarding how to prevent and treat it. What seems to be preventing these medical strides are severe missteps in the health community, thus leading what many believe is a lapsed response while causing more cases and ultimately, more deaths. Early on, when the coronavirus began to spread into parts of the community, it seemed to catch healthcare facilities by surprise. There was speculation that perhaps the Santa Clara county community was exposed to the virus a month before health officials knew. Compounding to this already alarming world event is the confusion that is occurring in hospitals.

There is simply not a reliable mitigation plan set up to accurately diagnose and track cases. Changing definitions of what constitutes a confirmed case of COVID-19, and overdiagnosis and misdiagnosis of the illness, makes it difficult to determine the real number of those affected.

Faulty Testing

One such misstep in question is the reliance on insufficient and unreliable tests to diagnose patients with COVID-19. Rather than using a coronavirus test kit provided by WHO, the CDC chose to create its own testing kit. When that kit was sent out to labs to confirm cases on-site, some were faulty and produced inconclusive results. In fact, reports suggest some people test negative up to six times even though they are infected with the virus. Flawed testing kits prevented local officials from taking a crucial first step in controlling the spread of the virus in communities. They are now weeks away from where they should be and the inevitability of viral hotspots has now become all the more real.

Another failed step was the strict criteria the CDC implemented on who could be tested. Only recent travelers from China or people who had contact with an infected person were tested, a move that health officials say failed to diagnose the early cases of the community spread virus in California and Washington state.

Perhaps, the most concerning is that epidemiologists have been unable to uncover a common denominator in patients, meaning how many people have actually been infected. That number will include people who never had symptoms or had a flu-like illness but never got a test for COVID-19. Until that vital information is uncovered, we are at the mercy of the virus.

Hospital Preparedness Plans

Keeping the logistical challenges in mind, hospitals and medical staff are preparing for a sudden surge of arriving patients and want to be ready to rapidly process a large number of casualties through the system. With the "whole-community emergency approach" previously mentioned including hospitals and healthcare systems, their work is cut out for them.

On average, 1 in 5 coronavirus patients require hospitalization due to the severe symptoms. If we see hospitalization numbers like we are currently seeing in Italy, you can easily guess how overwhelmed out medical system can become.

In a public press conference, Dr. Nancy Messonnier, director of Center for Disease Control and Prevention's National Center for Immunization and Respiratory Diseases, indicated that they have planned for coronavirus to stress hospitals. She states, "But as we project outward with the potential for this to be a much longer situation, one of the things that we're actively working on is projecting the long-term needs for our health care system."[7]

Hospitals are mobilizing resources and modifying protocols as new information about the virus emerges. Their plans are modified from what hospitals dealt with in past pandemics where they are prioritizing these main issues: identify, isolate, and inform. They understand the rapidly unfolding COVID-19 situation in the US could become more serious, with sustained community transmission, and is taking steps to make sure there are enough supplies and appropriate guidance to prevent spread of disease, especially among healthcare personnel caring for patients with COVID-19.

Their focus:

- Prevent the spread of respiratory diseases including COVID-19 within the facility
- Promptly identify and isolate patients with possible COVID-19 and inform the correct facility staff and public health authorities
- Care for a limited number of patients with confirmed or suspected COVID-19 as part of routine operations

- Potentially care for a larger number of patients in the context of an escalating outbreak
- Monitor and manage any healthcare personnel that might be exposed to COVID-19
- Communicate effectively within the facility and plan for appropriate external communication related to COVID-19

Containment Efforts

Once a contagion such as the novel coronavirus gets out in the open, mitigation efforts are a top priority. With such a high infection rate, a few hundred cases easily could turn into thousands and with that, a whole other problem occurs for the health care system—treatment centers. If this epidemic—and possibly pandemic—continues to infect large groups of the population, hospitals will face a bed shortage and have continued supply issues.

Across the US, hospitals are also modifying screening and triage protocols to detect COVID-19 patients as early as possible. Further, they are conducting drills on the identification, transport, rooming, and safe care of patients who may have been infected with COVID-19.

They are also focusing on containing the pathogen inside of a hospital setting by having and isolating airborne pathogens in an isolation room, properly maintaining ventilation systems, and using barriers such as glass/plastic windows in order to effectively reduce exposures to potentially infectious patients. But, without the proper protective equipment like respirators and disposable gowns due to high demand, they risk contracting the virus from those they are trying to help treat.

Bed Shortages

Just as the CDC is learning from previous pandemic events, our healthcare system is trying to learn from the current outbreak in the Wuhan Province. What healthcare providers have learned is how quickly cases soared in Wuhan and how fast they ran out of doctors and beds.

Experts warn the lethality of coronavirus will depend on how patients are cared for, treated, and, in particular, the availability of critical care beds. Given this virus is highly contagious, health experts would prefer COVID-19 diagnosed patients be in a room that prevents further contamination.

What Do I Do If I Become Sick With a Fast-Spreading Virus Like COVID-19?

If you are sick with COVID-19 or suspect you are infected with the virus that causes COVID-19, follow the steps below to help prevent the disease from spreading to people in your home and community. Here are the recommendations from the CDC on what you need to do.

Stay home except to get medical care: People who are mildly ill with COVID-19 are able to isolate at home during their illness. You should restrict activities outside your home, except for getting medical care. Do not go to work, school, or public areas. Avoid using public transportation, ride sharing, or taxis.

Separate yourself from other people and animals in your home:

People: As much as possible, you should stay in a specific room and away from other people in your home. Also, you should use a separate bathroom, if available.

Animals: You should restrict contact with pets and other animals while you are sick with COVID-19, just like you would around other people. Although there have not been reports of pets or other animals becoming sick with COVID-19, it is still recommended that people sick with COVID-19 limit contact with animals until more information is known about the virus. When possible, have another member of your household care for your animals while you are sick. If you are sick with COVID-19, avoid contact with your pet, including petting, snuggling, being kissed or licked, and sharing food. If you must care for your pet or be around animals while you are sick, wash your hands before and after you interact with pets and wear a facemask. See COVID-19 and Animals for more information.

Call ahead before visiting your doctor: If you have a medical appointment, call the healthcare provider and tell them that you have or may have COVID-19. This will help the healthcare provider's office take steps to keep other people from getting infected or exposed.

Wear a facemask: You should wear a facemask when you are around other people (e.g., sharing a room or vehicle) or pets and before you enter a healthcare provider's office. If you are not able to wear a facemask (for example, because it causes trouble breathing), then people who live with you should not stay in the same room with you, or they should wear a facemask if they enter your room.

Cover your coughs and sneezes: Cover your mouth and nose with a tissue when you cough or sneeze. Throw used tissues in a lined trash can. Immediately wash your hands with soap and water for at least 20 seconds or, if soap and water are not available, clean your hands with an alcohol-based hand sanitizer that contains at least 60% alcohol.

Clean your hands often: Wash your hands often with soap and water for at least 20 seconds, especially after blowing your nose, coughing, or sneezing; going to the bathroom; and before eating or preparing food. If soap and water are not readily available, use an alcohol-based hand sanitizer with at least 60% alcohol, covering all surfaces of your hands and rubbing them together until they feel dry.

Soap and water are the best option if hands are visibly dirty. Avoid touching your eyes, nose, and mouth with unwashed hands. The CDC offers these hand washing guidelines:[8]

Follow Five Steps to Wash Your Hands the Right Way

Washing your hands is easy, and it's one of the most effective ways to prevent the spread of germs. Clean hands can stop germs from spreading from one person to another and throughout an entire community—from your home and workplace to childcare facilities and hospitals.

Follow these five steps every time.

1. **Wet** your hands with clean, running water (warm or cold), turn off the tap, and apply soap.
2. **Lather** your hands by rubbing them together with the soap. Lather the backs of your hands, between your fingers, and under your nails.
3. **Scrub** your hands for at least 20 seconds. Need a timer? Hum the "Happy Birthday" song from beginning to end twice.
4. **Rinse** your hands well under clean, running water.
5. **Dry** your hands using a clean towel or air dry them.

Avoid sharing personal household items: You should not share dishes, drinking glasses, cups, eating utensils, towels, or bedding with other people or pets in your home. After using these items, they should be washed thoroughly with soap and water.

Clean all "high-touch" surfaces everyday: High touch surfaces include counters, tabletops, doorknobs, bathroom fixtures, toilets, phones, keyboards, tablets, and bedside tables. Also, clean any surfaces that may have blood, stool, or body fluids on them. Use a household cleaning spray or wipe, according to the label instructions. Labels contain instructions for safe and effective use of the cleaning product including precautions you should take when applying the product, such as wearing gloves and making sure you have good ventilation during use of the product.

Monitor your symptoms: Seek prompt medical attention if your illness is worsening (e.g., difficulty breathing). Before seeking care, call your healthcare provider and tell them that you have, or are being evaluated for, COVID-19. Put on a facemask before you enter the facility. These steps will help the healthcare provider's office to keep other people in the office or waiting room from getting infected or exposed. Ask your healthcare provider to call the local or state health department. Persons who are placed under active monitoring or facilitated self-monitoring should follow instructions provided by their local health department or occupational health professionals, as appropriate.

If you have a medical emergency and need to call 911, notify the dispatch personnel that you have, or are being evaluated for COVID-19. If possible, put on a facemask before emergency medical services arrive.

When to Discontinue Home Isolation

Patients with confirmed COVID-19 should remain under home isolation precautions until the risk of secondary transmission to others is thought to be low. The decision to discontinue home isolation precautions should be made on a case-by-case basis, in consultation with healthcare providers and state and local health departments.

Your Pandmic PPE Medical Essentials

Given the above missteps and concerns that the healthcare system has, we must assume that front line health care or medical response will collapse and will be overwhelmed, understaffed, and under-stocked in the event of a pandemic. Therefore, it is a real possibility that you and your loved ones will either take their chances at a temporary triage center or have to manage the illness at home.

Not only do you need to stockpile items for protecting yourself from a virulent disease, you need to know what happens if the worst-case scenario occurs and you or a loved one gets sick.

First and foremost, mimic what the healthcare professionals are doing during time of pandemic concerns. If the CDC is getting ready and recommending healthcare professionals to have personal protective equipment or PPE, then you should too! At the very least, here are some items they are recommending to healthcare professionals: Disposable gowns, gloves, NIOSH-certified disposable N95 respirator, and eye protection. Further, have a supply of medicines for respiratory illnesses, health-boosting vitamins, and foods.

The pandemic Personal Preparedness Equipment (PPE) essentials:

- Facemask
- Latex or nitrile disposable gloves
- Disposable surgical gown
- 60% Alcohol-based hand sanitizers

These are the basics of your PPE and should be used if you are around someone who is showing symptoms of a contagious pandemic illness. Remember, you want to protect your hands and cover your mouth and nose to stop yourself from touching your face and breathing in contaminated air particles. As a precaution, after touching, coming in contact with or leaving the sick room of someone who in contagious, after you remove your mask, gloves, or other protective equipment, wash your hands with soap and water thoroughly and then use hand sanitizer to keep hands clean.

In the following pages, we are going to break down each PPE essential so you fully understand their importance to your personal protection.

Facemask

While the CDC recommends wearing a face mask if you have COVID-19, are concerned someone around you is positive with the virus, or are caring for someone who is ill, it is equally as important to do as your conscience dictates.

Not all facemasks perform the same tasks so it is important to understand the options out there. There are different types of facemasks you should know about. This information is taken from OSHA and their *Guidance on Preparing Workplaces for an Influenza Pandemic.*[9]

Surgical masks: These masks are used as a physical barrier to protect employees from hazards such as splashes of large droplets of blood or body fluids. Surgical masks also prevent contamination by trapping large particles of body fluids that may contain bacteria or viruses when they are expelled by the wearer, thus protecting other people against infection from the person wearing the surgical mask.

Surgical/procedure masks are used for several different purposes, including the following:

- Placed on sick people to limit the spread of infectious respiratory secretions to others.
- Worn by healthcare providers to prevent accidental contamination of patients' wounds by the organisms normally present in mucus and saliva.
- Worn by employees to protect themselves from splashes or sprays of blood or body fluids; they may also have the effect of keeping contaminated fingers/hands away from the mouth and nose.

Surgical masks are not designed or certified to prevent the inhalation of small airborne contaminants. These small airborne contaminants are too little to see with the naked eye but may still be capable of causing infection.

Respirators: Respirators are designed to reduce an employee's exposure to airborne contaminants. Respirators are designed to fit the face and to provide a tight seal between the respirator's edge and the face. A proper seal between the user's face and the respirator forces inhaled air to be pulled through the respirator's filter material and not through gaps between the face and respirator.

- **Disposable or filtering facepiece respirators, where the entire respirator facepiece is comprised of filter material.** This type of respirator is also commonly referred to as an "N95" respirator. It is discarded when it becomes unsuitable for further use due to excessive breathing resistance (e.g., particulate clogging the filter, unacceptable contamination/soiling, or physical damage.).
- **Surgical respirators** are a type of respiratory protection that offers the combined protective properties of both a filtering facepiece respirator and a surgical mask. Surgical N95 respirators are certified by NIOSH as respirators and also cleared by FDA as medical devices which have been designed and tested and shown to be equivalent to surgical masks in certain performance characteristics (resistance to blood penetration, biocompatibility) which are not examined by NIOSH during its certification of N95 respirators.
- **Reusable or elastomeric respirators**, where the facepiece can be cleaned, repaired, and reused, but the filter cartridges are discarded and replaced when they become unsuitable for further use. These respirators come in half-mask (covering the mouth and nose) and full-mask (covering mouth, nose, and eyes) types. These respirators can be used with a variety of different cartridges to protect against different hazards. These

respirators can also be used with canisters or cartridges that will filter out gases and vapors.

- **Powered air purifying respirators (PAPRs)**, where a battery-powered blower pulls contaminated air through filters, then moves the filtered air to the wearer's facepiece. PAPRs are significantly more expensive than other air purifying respirators but they provide higher levels of protection and may also increase the comfort for some users by reducing the physiologic burden associated with negative pressure respirators and providing a constant flow of air on the face. These respirators can also be used with canisters or cartridges that will filter out gases and vapors. It should also be noted that there are hooded PAPRs that do not require employees to be fit tested in order to use them.

Facemask FAQs

When should you wear a mask?

The CDC recommends people who care for a pandemic flu patient at home or have other close contact with sick people in a pandemic to consider wearing an N-95 respirator.

If people are not able to avoid crowded places, large gatherings, or are caring for people who are ill, using a facemask or a respirator correctly and consistently could help protect people and reduce the spread of pandemic influenza.

Wear a mask if you are considered to be in an at-risk part of the population who may be more susceptible to the contagion and plan on traveling to an airport/flying on an airplane, or if you'll be amongst people in tight quarters.

Where can I find respirator masks?

N95 respirators can be found at home improvement stores like Lowe's or Home Depot, superstores like Walmart and

Target, Walgreens, CVS, wellness stores, and medical supply stores.

Can my child wear a N95 mask? What if I have facial hair?

N95 respirators are not designed for children or people with facial hair. A proper fit cannot be achieved on children. As well, those who have facial hair have a difficult time getting a full seal with an N95 respirator. Therefore, it may not provide the full protection a person is wanting.

What happens if my facemask is damaged?

If your mask is damaged or soiled, or if breathing through the mask becomes difficult, you should remove the face mask, discard it safely, and with clean hands, replace it with a new one. Be careful not to touch the filter portion of the mask. Try and put the mask on using the elastic loops. To safely discard your mask, place it in a plastic bag and put it in the trash. Wash your hands after handling the used mask.

Can I Reuse my disposable respirator?

Disposable respirators are designed to be used once and are then to be properly disposed of. Once worn in the presence of an infectious patient, the respirator should be considered potentially contaminated with infectious material, and touching the outside of the device should be avoided to prevent self-inoculation (touching the contaminated respirator and then touching one's eyes, nose, or mouth). It should be noted that a once-worn respirator will also be contaminated on its inner surface by the microorganisms present in the exhaled air and oral secretions of the wearer.

If a supply shortage occurs during a pandemic, employers and employees may consider reuse as long as the device has not been obviously soiled or damaged (e.g., creased or torn), and it retains its ability to function properly. This practice is not acceptable under normal circumstances and should only be considered under the most dire of conditions. Reuse may increase the potential for contamination; however, this risk must be balanced against the need to provide respiratory protection.

Follow these directions to re-use a facemask:

- Wear a clean set of gloves. Carefully, remove your N95 masks, laying it mouth-side down on a clean surface. Remove gloves.

- To re-use the mask: Wearing a new set of gloves, attempt to handle the mask only by the straps, and get it onto your face without contaminating yourself with the exterior touching your face. Avoid touching the eyes, mouth, and membranes of your nose. Your goal is to avoid the exterior of the mask coming into contact with anything that will transmit virus.

What You need to know about facemasks and N95 respirators

When the National Institute for Occupational Safety and Health (NIOSH) specified there be requirements for different respirator filters, they created three divisions for the filters with differing specifications: N series, R series, and P series. Using masks with air-purifying respirators protects by filtering particles out of the air the user is breathing. There are seven classes of filters for NIOSH-approved filtering facepiece respirators available at this time.

- N95 – Filters at least 95% of airborne particles. Not resistant to oil.

- Surgical N95 – A NIOSH-approved N95 respirator that has also been cleared by the Food and Drug Administration (FDA) as a surgical mask.

- N99 – Filters at least 99% of airborne particles. Not resistant to oil.

- N100 – Filters at least 99.97% of airborne particles. Not resistant to oil.
- R95 – Filters at least 95% of airborne particles. Somewhat resistant to oil.
- P95 – Filters at least 95% of airborne particles. Strongly resistant to oil.
- P99 – Filters at least 99% of airborne particles. Strongly resistant to oil.
- P100 – Filters at least 99.97% of airborne particles. Strongly resistant to oil.

The difference between the N-series, R-series, and P-series of masks has to do with whether or not the mask will be worn in an environment where oils and their vapors can be inhaled. In short, N-series filters are not resistant to oil, R-series filters are resistant to oil, and P-series filters are oil proof.

The respirator filter ratings (95, 99, 100) refer to the percentage efficiency at removing particulates from breathing air. 95, 99 and 100 series filters are 95%, 99% and 100% efficient, respectively.

N95 respirators made by different companies were found to have different filtration efficiencies for the most penetrating particle size (0.1 to 0.3 micron), but all were at least 95% efficient at that size. Above the most penetrating particle size, the filtration efficiency increases with size; it reaches approximately 99.5% or higher at about 0.75 micron. Tests with bacteria of size and shape similar to Mycobacterium tuberculosis also showed filtration efficiencies of 99.5% or higher.

Latex or nitrile disposable gloves

Wearing disposable gloves while out in public could create an important barrier between you and a pandemic contagion. It is essential for you to keep in mind the world you are living in now that there is a quickly spreading pandemic is different.

Health experts report that as much as 80% of infections are spread by hand contact. In times of pandemic outbreak, latex or nitrile gloves will block infectious germs from coming in contact directly with your hands. If you do not have gloves while out in a public setting or are concerned about surfaces having a contagious illness present, experts suggest using a tissue as barrier on public hard surfaces such as an escalator railing, elevator buttons, etc.

A pandemic is a life changing event. There is a contagious disease moving through the community and anytime you go outside, you are taking a gamble. Therefore, consider all outside surfaces to be contaminated. Wear gloves while out in public, using the gasoline pump, grocery shopping, and all other outside activities.

What the best type of disposable glove?

According to WHO, gloves used during an influenza outbreak should have these characteristics. The same would apply to the COVID-19 pandemic.

- Be nitrile, powder-free, non-sterile.
- Cuff length, preferably reaching mid forearm (eg. minimum 280mm total length. Sizes, S, M, L)
- Outer glove should have long cuffs, reaching well above the wrist, ideally to mid-forearm.
- Inner glove should be worn under the cuff of the gown/coveralls (and under any thumb/finger loop) whereas the outer glove should be worn over the cuff of the gown/coveralls.

Two-color glove system: the best way to double glove for optimum protection

At the time of the coronavirus scare, the WHO recommendation was one pair of gloves be worn by healthcare providers.

If you are concerned about risk of contamination from pinholes in gloves, consider the double glove system.

A best practice when double-gloving is to select a different color for each layer. This is because perforation of single gloves is often not detected during times of use. This increases the risk of blood-borne infections.

Incorporating a second color has two benefits:

- Double gloving significantly reduces the change of perforation
- If tearing does occur, it will be easier for the eye to spot

In situations where the top glove has ripped, it's best to replace both gloves for safety purposes.

How to Properly Remove Gloves

1. Pinch the outside of the glove about an inch or two down from the top edge inside the wrist.
2. Peel downwards, away from the wrist, turning the glove inside out
3. Pull the glove away until it's removed from the hand. Hold the inside-out glove with the gloved hand.
4. With your gloveless hand, slide your fingers under the wrist of the glove, do not touch the outside surface of the glove.
5. Repeat step 3. Peel downwards, away from the wrist, turning the glove inside out.
6. Continue pulling the glove down and over the first glove. This ensures that both gloves are inside out, one glove enveloped inside the other, with no contaminants on the bare hands.
7. Dispose of the gloves in a proper bin.
8. Proper hand hygiene should happen after glove disposal.

Disposable gowns

Wear a disposable gown when it is anticipated that soiling of clothes or uniform with blood or other bodily fluids, including respiratory secretions, may occur. Most routine pandemic COVID-19 patient encounters do not necessitate the use of gowns.

Isolation gowns can be disposable and made of synthetic material or reusable and made of washable cloth. Gowns should be the appropriate size to fully cover the areas requiring protection. After patient care is performed, the gown should be removed and placed in a laundry receptacle or waste container, as appropriate. Hand hygiene should follow.

Alternatively, a Tyvek suit will also provide adequate protection against biological agents from a pandemic. As well, they can be used in tandem with a respirator. These suits are considered limited-use and are made of spunste polyethylene and are made to keep particulate matter and light oil and liquid away from the wearer.

How to clean reusable suits

To clean a Tyvek or reusable suit, simply hand wash with mild soap (no bleach) or machine wash, gentle cycle, cold water. Drip dry only. Do not put in a dryer, dry clean, or use an iron on this fabric.

Alcohol-Based Sanitizer

While hand washing with soap and water for at least 20 seconds is recommended, especially after going to the bathroom, before eating, and after blowing your nose, coughing, or sneezing,if soap and water are not readily available, use a hand sanitizer that contains at least 60% alcohol. Always wash your hands with soap and water if your hands are visibly dirty.

Alcohol-based hand sanitizer is a must for pandemic preparations. It is just another way to keep hands free of germs and nasty pathogens. When using a hand sanitizer that uses 60 percent isopropyl alcohol, its antimicrobial properties kill 99.9% of the bacteria on hands 30 seconds after application and 99.99% to 99.999% in one minute. As well, it has the ability to denature proteins. The only viruses they do not kill are some common germs such as salmonella, e. Coli, MRSA (methicillin-resistant Staphylococcus aureus), and norovirus.

Stock up on alcohol-based hand sanitizers. If you can't find any, make them.

Note: Do not rinse or wipe off the hand sanitizer before it's dry; it may not work as well against germs.

Washing Hands vs. Hand Sanitizer

There are important differences between washing hands with soap and water and cleaning them with hand sanitizer. For example, alcohol-based hand sanitizers don't kill ALL types of germs, such as a stomach bug called norovirus, some parasites, and Clostridium difficile, which causes severe diarrhea. Hand sanitizers also may not remove harmful chemicals, such as pesticides and heavy metals like lead.

Handwashing for twenty seconds or longer reduces the amounts of all types of germs, pesticides, and metals on hands. Knowing when to clean your hands and which method to use will give you the best chance of preventing sickness.

Pandemic Medical Supplies for the Home

A month's supply of medicine is vital for anyone under quarantine or caring for someone at home. Since many pharmaceutical drugs are manufactured in China, the origin of Coronavirus, drug shortages could become even more pronounced during a pandemic, which could cut off pharmaceutical supply chains in various parts of the world.

The Department of Homeland Security advises US citizens to prepare copies and electronic versions of their health records and pharmacies. See about ordering a month's worth of prescription medications in case the supply chain becomes disrupted and there is a shortage. If your local pharmacy does not have them, order online. You do not want to take the chance of not having vital prescription medicines during a pandemic.

Essential medical items to have in place are:

- any prescription drugs
- pain relievers
- stomach remedies
- cough and cold medicines
- fluids with electrolytes
- vitamins

A power packed natural approach to vitamins

Finding the right supplements can be a tricky endeavor. But what if I told you it doesn't have to be? In fact, you could easily grow your own vitamins naturally from the convenience of your kitchen window. What am I talking about? I'm talking about sprouts.

Sprouts are nature's multivitamin and provide the highest amount of vitamins, minerals, proteins, and enzymes of any of food per unit of calorie. They are commonly referred to as a complete food because they are packed with high levels of complete proteins, vitamins, minerals, enzymes, and extraordinary amounts of protein. And they're cheap!

How do spouts benefit the body? Consuming sprouts will:

- Assist in healing the body
- Cleanse the body
- Help prevent diseases
- Enhance the general functioning of bodily organs
- Aid in digestion
- Remove gas from the stomach

Some of the most popular types of seeds to sprout are mung beans, alfalfa, broccoli, beets, hard red wheat, radish, sweet pea, and carrot seeds. Try and stay away from the nightshade family of seeds such as eggplants and tomatoes. They contain an alkaloid called solanine (present in potatoes too), which is toxic in high concentrations.

Almost anything can be made into a sprout! The most common types of seeds to sprout include alfalfa, grains, peas, lentils, radish, broccoli, cabbage, mustard seed, garbanzos, quinoa, nuts, and red clover. Sprouts can be grown every week for continuous staggered batches. In fact, there are sprout kits available to help you expand your sprouting palate.

1. First, you need something to let your seeds sprout in. If you have a large mason jar, that will work too. We like adding a sprouting lid to the top of our mason jar sprouts to help with easy rinsing. If you plan on sprouting different varieties of sprouts, you may want to invest in a low-cost four-tray sprouting kit. For large seeds, like beans and legumes, consider adding them to a large wide-mouth jar. When beans begin to sprout, they will quickly take up a lot of room. For smaller seeds, using a quart-sized jar or the sprouting tray would work well.

2. Next, you need to right kind of seeds. Purchase sprouting seeds that are non-GMO and organic varieties to avoid seeds that are chemically treated.

3. Now that you have your vessel and seeds picked out, it's time to start sprouting. Simply add a tablespoon or two of seeds in a jar and fill it about ¾ full with cool water. Swish the seeds around and allow the water to drain from the jar or sprouting tray. Once the water has drained, cover with a mesh lid or cloth, secured with a rubber band, to allow air flow. Sprouting Tip: For larger beans like garbanzo or mung beans, allow them to soak

overnight and then drain the water in the morning. Repeat the rinsing step twice a day for 3–4 days.

4. Set sprouts in an area in the kitchen where they will receive indirect sunlight. Ideally, sprouts prefer a temperature of about 65-80ºF. If the temperature is warmer with increased humidity, rinse sprouts more frequently.

5. When sprouts are ready and have grown to the desired size, do a final rinse and drain them completely. They can be eaten immediately or transferred to a clean glass or plastic container and stored in the refrigerator for a few days. As a precaution, make sure the sprouts have drained completely before storing.

Sprout Safety: One of the biggest drawbacks to sprouting is their very short shelf life. Unlike other fresh produce, seeds and beans need warm and humid conditions to sprout and grow. These conditions are also ideal for the growth of bacteria, including Salmonella, Listeria, and E. coli. Not to cause concern, but since 1996, there have been at least 30 reported outbreaks of foodborne illness associated with different types of raw and lightly cooked sprouts. Most of these outbreaks were caused by Salmonella and E. coli and occurred at growing facilities. The bacteria are usually present in or on the seed, and the bacteria can grow to high levels during sprouting, even under sanitary conditions at home.

To prevent this health issue, you can follow these safety steps:

*   Wash all sprouts thoroughly with filtered water before eating them.
*   If you've purchased sprouts at the grocery store, look for the International Sprout Growers Association seal on the package or if you are buying bulk, ask your grocer if the sprouts are ISGA-approved.

- If the sprouts are pre-packaged, only purchase if the sell-by date is current or even a few days ahead.
- Examine the sprouts to make sure the roots are clean. If the stem color is not white or creamy, do not purchase them. Do not purchase sprouts if the buds are no longer attached if they are dark in color or have a musty smell.
- Smell the sprouts to be sure that they have a clean, fresh odor.
- Keep the sprouts refrigerated.
- After 2 days, compost them rather than consuming them yourself.
- If you're buying in bulk, ask your grocer about the sell-by date.
- If you are sprouting seeds at home, follow the same guidelines described above. Learn about the source of your seeds, their ISGA-certification, and either have your grocer confirm high-quality standards for seed production or obtain contact information for the seed source and contact that company yourself.
- Follow the above guidelines regardless of the type of seeds you are sprouting, i.e., apply the guidelines to mung, alfalfa, radish, broccoli, lentil, sunflower and all other types of sprouts.

Since the shelf life is around 2 days before the sprouts begin to break down, take advantage of having them and add them to salads, sandwiches, soups, and even bread for added nutrition.

Future antibiotic shortages

Another overlooked medical supply briefly touched on in this guide and one that many often forget about when they are wanting to prepare for pandemics are lifesaving antibiotics. Many fail to realize that antibiotic shipments may become affected during pandemic scares and shortages in the product can occur. Raw materials from China that are used for pharmaceutical drugs including antibiotics like penicillin may not be available if there's an interruption in the supply chain. Your doctor may be able to write you a prescription or, alternatively you can consider fish antibiotics. While it is not recommended for humans, in an emergency situation, you have a choice to make if your life is on the line.

Fish antibiotics have been popular amongst preppers because no prescription is required to purchase them. It is true many fish antibiotics contain the same active ingredients as those formulated for humans. However, there are a few considerations to keep in mind, such as using the correct dosage as to not over medicate yourself, and the differences in human metabolism vs. the metabolism rate of a fish. Anyone who is planning on storing up fish antibiotics to use needs to do proper research.

- FISH-MOX (amoxicillin 250 mg)
- FISH_MOX FORTE (amoxicillin 500 mg)
- FISH-CILLIN (ampicillin 250 mg)
- FISH-FLEX Keflex 250 mg)
- FISH-FLEX FORTE (Keflex 500 mg)
- FISH-ZOLE (metronidazole 250 mg)
- FISH-PEN (penicillin 250 mg)
- FISH-PEN FORTE (penicillin 500 mg)
- FISH-CYCLINE (tetracycline 250 mg)

NOTE: It should be emphasized FISH-CYCLINE [and other tetracycline antibiotics of various names] can become toxic after its expiration date, unlike most of the other medications listed.

These medications are available usually in plastic bottles of 100 tablets for much less than the same prescription medication at the pharmacy (some come in bottles of 30 tablets). The dosages are similar to that used in humans, and are taken two to four times a day, depending on the drug. The 500mg dosage is probably more effective in larger individuals. Of course, anyone could be allergic to one or another of these antibiotics, but not all of them. (Note there is a 10% cross-reactivity between "-cillin" drugs and Keflex, meaning, if you are allergic to Penicillin, you could also be allergic to Keflex). FISH-ZOLE is an antibiotic that also kills some protozoa that cause dysentery.

Antibiotics are an essential preparedness item to have on hand for extended disasters; however, they should only be taken when they are needed the most. Understanding the differences between the different antibiotic families, knowing the effects they can have on the body, as well as knowing which antibiotics would be best for specific medical conditions will help you make the right choice when comes to buying them. Certain antibiotics should not be mixed with other drugs, foods, or alcohol. Therefore, consult a doctor before taking antibiotics.

Build the Ultimate One-Year Medical Supply

Experts suggest that each home has a basic medical supply that is unique to your family's needs. It is in your best interest to ensure that you have any and all necessary medications that require prescriptions before an emergency happens.

We all have our fair share of band-aids and antibiotic ointment, but do you have medical supplies that can help with true medical emergencies? The following list is your basic medical preparations broken into sections of need to help in your organization.

Hygiene

- Liquid antibacterial hand soap – 20 bottles
- Disposable hand wipes – 20 packages
- Antibacterial hand sanitizer – 20 containers
- Feminine items – 12 packages

- Extra baby needs (diapers, wipes, pacifiers, bottles, medicine, etc.) – in quantity

- Disposable Nitrile gloves – 5 boxes or more

Essential Medical Tools

- Trauma shears
- Penlight or small flashlight
- Scalpel with extra blades
- Stethoscope

- Irrigation syringe
- Tweezers
- Thermometer
- Foam splint – 2 per family member
- Thermometer

Over-the-Counter Products

- Aspirin or non-aspirin pain reliever (for adults and children) – 5 bottles
- Stool softener – 5 bottles
- Electrolyte powder – 3 boxes
- Cold/flu medications – 3 boxes per family member
- Expectorant/decongestants – 3 per family member

- Hydrocortisone – 3 tubes
- Miconazole/anti-fungal – 3 tubes or spray bottles
- Syrup of Ipecac and activated charcoal – 2 containers
- Eye care (e.g., contact lens case, cleansing solution, eye moisture drops) – 3 per family member

Natural Supplements

- Potassium iodide tablets – 1 box per family member
- Multivitamins – 2 large containers

- Vitamin C – 1-2 large containers
- Ginger – 1 bottle
- Garlic – 1 bottle or grow your own
- Ginseng – 2 bottles

- Colloidal silver – 1 container per family member

Wound Care

- Disinfectant (Betadine, isopropyl alcohol, iodine, hydrogen peroxide, etc.) – 2 per family member
- Band-aids – 3 large boxes in assorted sizes
- Antibiotic ointment – 5
- Instant cold and hot packs – 10
- 1 week of prescription medications – as many as you are able to get with your prescription
- Ace bandages – 10
- Non- stick gauze pads in assorted sizes (3×3 and 4×4) – 10 boxes
- Sterile roller bandages – 5

- Surgical sponges – 5
- Adhesive tape or duct tape – 5
- Steri-strips – 5
- Moleskin – 3
- Respirator masks – 4 cases for short-term events. For longer-term events multiply the supply.
- CPR micro shield – 1 per family member
- Suture kit – 3 per family member
- QuikClot® compression bandages – 2 per family member
- Tourniquet – 2
- Thermal Mylar blanket – 1 per family member
- Antibiotics – 2 types per family member

Storing Medical Supplies

How you store your first aid supplies is every bit as important as having the supplies in the first place. Medicines can lose potency or spoil if they are subject to moisture, temperature fluctuations, and light. For example, aspirin begins to break down when it is exposed to a slight amount of moisture.

Unless the instructions indicate otherwise, store medications in a cool, dark place that is out of the reach of children. However, you still want to store the medical supplies in a place that is easily accessible to adults, who may need to respond very quickly in the event of a medical crisis.

Check expiration dates periodically to ensure the medicines are still good to use. While most medicines lose potency once they're past the expiration date, there are a few that will actually make a person extremely ill if taken after it spoils. For example, tetracycline antibiotics that have spoiled can cause a severe, sometimes deadly, kidney ailment.

Signs of expired medicines

Although there is data that states most medicines can last longer than their expiration dates, it is important to understand that medicine years past its expiration date can lose effectiveness and in some cases, change its chemical makeup. If you are in a survival situation where your life depended on an outdated drug, then it is wise to follow the cliché "better safe than sorry."

Knowing the signs of expired medicine can help indicate when new items are needed.

- Creams or ointments which are discolored or have changed in texture.
- Creams or ointments which have cracked or separated.
- The medicine's smell has changed since it was opened.
- Tablets are broken or chipped and have changed color.

Bear in mind, there are some medications that should never be used after their expiration and could have severe consequences for patients. These include:

- Anticonvulsants – narrow therapeutic index
- Dilantin, phenobarbital – very quickly lose potency

- Nitroglycerin – very quickly lose potency
- Warfarin – narrow therapeutic index
- Procan SR – sustained release procainamide
- Theophylline – very quickly lose potency
- Digoxin – narrow therapeutic index
- Thyroid preparations
- Paraldehyde
- Oral contraceptives
- Epinephrine – very quickly lose potency
- Insulin – very quickly lose potency
- Eye drops – eyes are particularly sensitive to any bacteria that might grow in a solution once a preservative degrades.

What if you don't have enough medical supplies?

Now, let's take this a step further. What if you prepared your food and water for an emergency, but completely forgot about getting medical supplies? (It's hard to remember everything when you're planning for a disaster.) There are some alternatives that you may be lucky enough to have in your pantry to use.

Some of your kitchen staples may have some medicinal value. For instance, did you know you can make an antiseptic (first discovered during World War I) made of a diluted solution of baking soda and bleach? It's called Dakin's Solution and has been proven to kill most bacteria and viruses. As well, vinegar, baking soda, baking powder, and salt have medicinal values.

Uses for Dakin's Solution include minor scrapes and skin and tissue infections. It can be used before and after surgical procedures to prevent infection, can be used as a mouth wash (should not be swallowed), used as a wound irrigator solution to clean wounds, or can be applied as a wet-to-moist dressing for wounds.

Dakin's Solution

Supplies:
- Clean tap water
- Sterile measuring cups and spoons
- Clean pan with lid
- Baking soda
- Sodium hydrochlorite solution at 5.25% (Bleach, unscented)
- Sterile jar with a sterile lid
- Label for jar to label antiseptic, date, time and discard date

Instructions:
1. Wash your hands well with soap and water.
2. Measure out 32 ounces (4 cups) of clean water. Pour into a clean pan and allow water to boil for 15 minutes. Remove pan from heat.
3. Using a sterile measuring spoon, add 1/2 tsp. of baking soda to the water.
4. Measure the bleach according to the strength that is desired:
5. – For full strength – add 3 oz. bleach or 95 ml.
   – For 1/2 strength – add 3 tbls. + 1/2 tsp. or 48 ml.
   – For 1/4 strength – add 1 tbls. +2 tsp. or 24 ml.
   – For 1/8 strength – add 2 1/2 tsp. or 12-14 ml.
6. Place the solution in a jar and close it tightly with a sterile lid. Cover the closed jar with tin foil to protect it from sunlight.
7. Throw away any unused portion of the antiseptic within 48 hours of use. This solution can be made up to a month prior to using and stored away.

Health

Your immune system is another important part of your preparedness plan to consider and it's one of the most important because it's your last of defenses. Boosting your immune system can help you avoid becoming sick or reduce the severity of illness should you become infected. Practicing other good health habits, such as getting plenty of rest, exercising, drinking plenty of fluids, and managing stress, also can help stop the spread of germs and prevent the flu.

Make your own Vitamin C powder

You can easily make vitamin C using the biproduct of our favorite citrus fruits. Any organic citrus peel will work.

1. Wash and dry fruit. Slice or grate citrus peel. I usually grate my peels with a microplane grater and allow it to sit in a window for a few days. If you cut your peels into long strips, you can also use a dehydrator and the heat from the dehydrator will not harm the enzymes. This method is also ideal if you want to store your dried peels in a closed canning jar for longer-term storage for up to 1 year.
2. When you are ready to use your dried peels, break up peels into smaller pieces. If the peels are large, break apart and use a coffee grinder. If the peels are small enough, use a mortar and pestle to powder the peels.
3. Use 1 rounded teaspoon for a daily supply of organic vitamin C complex, rutin, hesperidin, and bioflavonoids that your body needs for the day, regardless of your size.
4. To use citrus peel powder:
5. Add 1 rounded teaspoon to your favorite beverage, smoothie, or on top of salads. Caution: Be careful about adding this powder to hot drinks or meals as the extreme heat destroys the beneficial enzymes.

Herbs, Natural Remedies, and Viral Pandemics

It is important to emphasize that herbs cannot cure a highly contagious virus, but they can certainly help boost your immunity. Turning toward natural remedies now will give you the knowledge and skills you need to keep your family well during flu season and in the event of a pandemic flu.

When you begin feeling that your body is run down, it is time to start actively working to boost the immune system. By doing so, you are fighting off the infection before it overtakes your body, thus significantly reducing being prone to colds and flu. You can help give your body the edge by trying the following:

- **Herbal Tinctures** – Herbal tinctures are natural medicines that help with a variety of ailments. You can stimulate your immune system function to help shorten the physical and mental recovery periods of illnesses. Herbal tinctures that support immune function include medicinal mushroom tinctures, Echinacea root tincture, elderberry tinctures, or lomatium root tinctures.
- **Teas** – Herbal teas can also help boost your immune system. You can help fortify your immune system during cold and flu season. Finding teas that have bioactive ingredients like echinacea, yarrow, lemon balm, elderberry, and marshmallow help you feel better naturally! Drinking any warm liquid calms our nerves, lowers our stress levels, and decreases blood pressure, as warmth itself is associated with comfort. As warm beverages also beg to be sipped as opposed to chugged quickly, it often means the person consuming the warm drink will be sitting down, calm, possibly reading, or just enjoying the quiet. This also helps boost the body's natural defense.
- **Sleep** – Getting enough quality sleep helps the body keep functioning at its best. I know when I don't get enough sleep, I feel worse than if I had a cold! If you

have trouble sleeping, try to look into ways to calm down before bed, such as drinking the aforementioned tea or exhausting yourself with exercise. Try to avoid alcohol, tobacco, and caffeine in the few hours before you go to bed. These vices all play a role in our sleeping habits, and not in a positive way. Caffeine and coffee can be amazing for the body, however, it definitely should be avoided before bed, unless you drink decaf.

- **Probiotics** – These teeny microorganisms help keep your gut running the way it should. Try eating more fermented foods. Fermented foods like kimchi, kefir, and kombucha are widely available these days. They give your body a healthy dose of probiotics, which are live microorganisms that are important to good digestion and overall health.
- **Elixirs** – Taking a daily teaspoon of an elixir can increase the immune system. Here are some of my favorites:

Homemade elixirs help the medicine go down

Elixirs like these recipes are an effective way to provide preventive medicine to your body and boost your health in the process. In fact, the health benefits of these ingredients for treating respiratory problems are unmatched.

Homemade Elderberry Syrup

- 2/3 cup black elderberries
- 3 1/2 cups water
- 2 tablespoons fresh or dried ginger root
- 1 teaspoon cinnamon powder
- 1/2 teaspoon cloves or clove powder
- 2 lemon or orange slices
- 3/4 cup raw honey

1. Pour water into medium saucepan and add elderberries, ginger, cinnamon, cloves, and citrus slices and

bring to a boil. Then, cover and reduce to a simmer for about 45 minutes to an hour until the liquid has reduced by almost half.

2. Remove from heat and let mixture cool enough to be handled. Pour through a strainer into a glass jar or bowl.

3. Discard the elderberries (or compost them!) and let the liquid cool to lukewarm. When it is no longer hot, add 3/4 cup of honey and stir well.

4. When honey is well mixed into the elderberry mixture, pour the syrup into a pint sized mason jar or 16 ounce glass bottle of some kind.

5. Ta Da! You just made homemade elderberry syrup! Store in the fridge and take daily for its immune boosting properties. Some sources recommend taking only during the week and not on the weekends to boost immunity.

6. Standard dose is 1/2 tsp to 1 tsp for kids and 1/2 Tbsp to 1 Tbsp for adults. If illness does strike, take the normal dose every 2–3 hours instead of once a day until symptoms disappear.

Homemade Slippery Elm Cough Elixir

- 3 1/2 cups filtered water
- 2 tablespoons slippery elm bark
- 1 tablespoon marshmallow root
- 2 tablespoons ginger root
- 2–3-inch piece cinnamon bark
- 1/3 cup elderberry for added immune boosting properties, optional
- 1/2 organic orange, sliced
- 1/2 cup local honey

1. Combine all dry herbal ingredients to the water and heat over medium heat (excluding orange slices and honey)

2. Bring mixture to a boil and reduce heat to a simmer for 30 minutes or until the liquid is reduced by half.
3. Remove the mixture from heat and allow to thoroughly cool.
4. Using a fine mesh sieve, strain liquid into a wide-mouth jar before stirring in honey.
5. Pack with orange slices and store in the fridge for up to one month.
  * A dose is 2 teaspoons up to 4 times a day.

Immune-Boosting Lemon, Honey, and Ginger Cough Syrup

- 2 to 3 lemons, sliced
- 3 tablespoons fresh ginger, peeled and coarsely chopped
- Honey

1. Wash lemons and cut into slices or wedges. Remove seeds and pack the wedges in a clean, dry 8-ounce Mason jar.
2. Peel and cut ginger root. Add 1 1/2 tablespoons into the jar with the lemon wedges.
3. Fill the jar with honey.
4. Close the jar and let stand for at least 24 hours before using.
5. Store in refrigerator or dark, cool pantry for up to 2 months.

More ways to boost your immunity

- **Get More Sun** – Sunlight triggers the skin's production of vitamin D. In the summer, 10–15 minutes of exposure (minus sunscreen) is enough. However, above 42 degrees latitude (Boston) from November through February, sunlight is too weak and very few foods contain adequate levels of this essential vitamin. Low vitamin D levels correlate with a greater risk of respiratory infection. A 2010 study in kids showed that 1200 IU a day of supplemental vitamin D reduced the risk of influenza A. This vitamin is essential to managing stress, which can also weaken your immune system.

- **Fast** – While most trendy cold and flu treatments involve consuming popular superfoods (some of which do have merit) it turns out that fasting, or abstaining from food, can help keep you from getting sick in the first place. Fasting for three days causes your immune system to completely regenerate. It prompts your body to start eliminating damaged immune cells and to start generating new more efficient cells. After three days without food, your immune system is completely rebuilt from the ground up, which is helpful for anyone with a damaged immune system, such as the elderly or cancer patients.

- **Spirulina** – This blue-green algae has been shown to have an effect on the immune system as well as having a detoxifying effect on the body. It also is rich in protein, vitamins, minerals, carotenoids, and antioxidants that can help protect cells from damage. Not bad for a little green powder!

- **Apple Cider Vinegar Tonic** – Apple cider vinegar has a fairly lengthy history when it comes to natural home remedies. It has been touted as a cure-all for almost everything, from helping blood pressure issues, fungal infections, to sore throats and even weight loss. And, because most germs can't survive in the overly acidic environment, it's perfect to take as an immune booster.

Apple Cider Vinegar Tonic

- 4 cups filtered water
- 2 tablespoons unfiltered apple cider vinegar (with mother)
- 3 tablespoons raw honey
- 2-inch piece fresh ginger chopped finely
- 1 cinnamon stick
- 1/2 lemon, juiced

6. In a large pitcher, combine all ingredients and refrigerate overnight.
7. Pour tonic in a small juice cup and enjoy once a day.

- **Honey –** This is already in your pantry and has become a poster child for an alternative to antibiotics. Itcan fight multiple species of bacteria, fungi, and superbugs. Honey is also good for wounds/abrasions/cuts of the mouth, as it is a demulcent that soothes abraded tissues, and it also is a medium that microbes do not live in. Who doesn't remember the time-honored honey and lemon mixture for a sore throat? The thing of it is, it works, and if it works it should be employed.
- **Mushrooms –** These have a profound healing effect on the body and are an untapped medicinal food source thanks to the polysaccharides in mushrooms. Polysaccharides, also known as beta-glucans, are similar to immune-boosting powers found in the medicinal plants of echinacea, and astragalus. They say the larger these beta glucans are, the stronger they are on the immune system. More notably, certain mushrooms, such as shiitake and reishi mushrooms, have antiviral and antibiotic properties.

- **Bone broth** – You want to give your body what it needs to stay as healthy as possible. Bone broth is a healing dietary staple our ancestors regularly consumed, along with fermented foods. Bone broth can aid in digestion, contains minerals that are easily absorbed, and is great for the immune system. Bone marrow helps the immune system by carrying oxygen to cells in the body.
- **Avoid bad habits** – Smoking cigarettes, vaping, drinking, and drug use can decrease your body's immunity to disease. As stressful and fearful as this time is, it's best not to partake in any bad habits. You want to do everything you can to keep your body at its maximum health.
- **Drink lots of water** – Simply put, water helps to filter the impurities out of your body. Over time, this keeps your body functioning and in optimum health.
- **Take your vitamins** – Vitamins A, B, C, D, and E have been shown to promote a healthy immune system. Take a high quality, organic multi-vitamin. Vitamin C and Zinc, in particular, are helpful immunity boosters. Since our bodies do not naturally make Vitamin C, we need to get it through supplementation in order to boost our bone, muscle, cartilage, and vascular health. The best way to get vitamin C is right from the source. Rather than taking a GMO vitamin, make your own vitamin C powder (see page xx).
- **Herbs** – Having access to health-inducing herbs is another essential for wound care. Herbs such as oregano, garlic, lavender, and thyme can help protect a wound from infection and promote healing. Further, knowing which herbs can be used for natural pain killers is paramount in your medical preparedness knowledge. Some pain reducing herbs to add to your herbal first-aid kit are:
  - Aloe (Aloe vera)
  - Calendula (Calendula officinalis)

- Comfrey (Symphytum officinale)
- Gotu Kola (Centella asiatica)
- Tea (Camellia sinensis)
- Lavender (Lavandula angustifolia)

Common pantry items can also be used to help bleeding wounds clot. Many have found that cayenne pepper is an effective alternative and natural version of QuikClot. Cayenne pepper contains an active ingredient, called capsaicin, which has analgesic (pain relieving) properties and various other medicinal uses.

Sanitation, good hygiene, and medical preparedness all go hand-in-hand. This multi-pronged approach can help keep you safe, protected, and healthy.

CHAPTER 5

How to Prepare the Home for a Pandemic

When a sudden disease takes hold of a community and then spreads infecting more communities, and then states, etc., it is alarming to say the least. As more cases are confirmed and health officials acknowledge there is a problem, people will panic. This is a given.

With the COVID-19 outbreak, after a handful of confirmed cases, we're already seeing shortages of pandemic prevention supplies such as respirator masks and full-body coveralls, hand sanitizers, paper goods like toilet paper and paper towels. If there is an escalation in cases and a pandemic disease continues to spread to more cities across America, you should fully expect a run on essential supplies like food, gas and bottled water.

Some will continue to believe this is under control; and maybe it will be soon. But what if it isn't? Are you prepared to take that risk by not developing a contingency plan that takes very little effort and can be done on a budget?

So just how do we prepare for this pandemic?

A big concern with pandemics is that supplies in stores would be quickly exhausted leaving many unprepared to handle the ordeal. This will only fuel a more chaotic situation. These concerns are not new to most governments and steps have been taken to ensure communities are prepared and able to contain most epidemics. That said, at a pandemic level, it is another story. There is a sense of urgency to be prepared before "the midnight hour." They creates extreme stress to those who are unprepared to handle even a three day emergency let alone one they are being advised to prepare for two weeks.

Which such a large-scale emergency, it is difficult to know where to start and the best answer this author can give you is to start preparedness efforts at home. We cannot control if or when a government will decide to prepare, but we can control when and what we, as individuals, need to protect our families. In fact, when it comes to pandemic preparedness, the government firmly believes in individual preparedness.

> The critical role of individuals and families in controlling a pandemic cannot be overstated. The success or failure of infection control measures is ultimately dependent upon the acts of individuals – practicing hand hygiene, cough etiquette, remaining home if ill or if a household member is ill, and complying with social distancing measures. The collective response of all Americans will be crucial in mitigating the health, social, and economic impacts of a pandemic. Everyone has a role to play in getting ready and staying healthy"
> —*The National Strategy for Pandemic Influenza*

Inform Yourself

The best defense against a pandemic virus is to avoid misinformation and panic (despite the understandable temptation to voraciously read everything, regardless of the source). Having first-hand knowledge of what pandemics are, how they behave, the government's protocols, and how the medical system plans to provide care can help you put together a solid plan and stay ahead of the game. Understanding that our lives will change drastically if the population is faced with a pandemic and being prepared for this can help you mentally prepare and make better choices toward the wellbeing of your family. Some assumed pandemic impacts are the following:

- Susceptibility to the pandemic virus will be universal.
- Once sustained person-to-person transmission begins, the disease will spread rapidly around the globe.
- Rates of absenteeism will depend on the severity of the pandemic. In a severe influenza pandemic, for example, absenteeism attributable to illness, the need to care for ill family members, and fear of infection may reach 40 percent during the peak weeks of a community outbreak.
- Epidemics will last 6–8 weeks in affected communities.
- Pandemics are multi-phasic meaning there would be multiple waves (periods where community outbreaks strike across the country) will likely occur with each lasting 2–3 months.
- Challenges or shutdowns of business commerce.
- Breakdown of our basic infrastructure: communications, mass transportation, supply chains
- Closing of banks or payroll service interruptions.
- Staffing shortages in hospitals and medical clinics.
- Interruptions in public facilities: Schools and workplaces may close, and public gatherings such as sporting events or worship services may close temporarily.
- Government mandated voluntary or involuntary home quarantine.

Supply disruptions for everyday living items could cause a nightmare situation for you and your family. When the demand is high to purchase specific items (such as preparedness items before or during a disaster), certain items sell out quickly. Keeping up with the desperate and immediate demands of hundreds of thousands of people will undoubtedly be a challenge in and of itself and supply trucks can only do so much, especially during unexpected times of pandemic outbreaks.

To make matters worse, if grocery stores run out of essential items in more population dense areas, those who cannot get what they need will drive to the smaller towns and take supplies from that store. The situation may become more dire if the grocery stores can put limits on how much you can buy. Looting and mayhem may follow suit.

It's important to know what you are facing—a fast-moving contagious disease and a mob of scared people with the same thing on their minds: "I've got to get prepared before it spreads!" Now it is time to put together your own personal preparedness plans. Do not wait until the last minute and take the chance of being left empty-handed. Those living in this aftermath have a long road ahead of them, and knowing which items disappear off the shelves first can help them better prepare and stay on top of their personal supplies.

But before you go out and purchase necessary supplies, it is important to prepare the home.

Preparing the Home

Preparing your home for the possibility of living through short or long-term quarantine measures and ensuring the home is a healthy environment that will support the wellbeing of you and your family will give you peace of mind. Let's get started.

During times of pandemics, it will be necessary to clean your home more frequently. Simply put, germs live on dirty surfaces and travel in dust particles, further infecting the home. Using spray disinfectants or bleach water can help remove germs including bacteria and viruses from dirty surfaces.

While many have concerns about tracking a contagious disease into the home, according to the CDC, that risk is still low. For example, many feared that COVID0-19 could be spread this way, but according to studies, the COVID-19 virus doesn't live long on soft fabrics like carpets and rugs, or even clothing. However, there is a concern with that particular virus being on hard surfaces like doorknobs, stair railings, and hands, etc.

Keeping this in mind, here are eight immediate steps you can take to prevent the spread of germs in your house.

1. Clean the dirtiest surfaces in your home: It's time to start doing this more regularly, since many of us are worried about the coronavirus.
2. The CDC recommends using gloves and disinfecting areas where there can be large numbers of household germs and where there is a possibility that these germs could be spread to others. Here are some hotspots to hit: doorknobs, faucet handles, toilet flushers, bathrooms, phones, keyboards, remote controls, countertops, and tables.
3. If you have children, sanitize hard plastic toys, especially if your child has been sick. Kids carry a lot of germs, and because of that, their immune systems are much stronger than ours. However, you don't want grandma getting sick after playing with the little ones.
4. Take your shoes off at the door. While this is not necessarily pandemic prevention, it will prevent tracking germs into the house. Did you know that E. coli was detected on 27% of shoes, along with seven other kinds of bacteria, including Klebsiella pneumoniae, which can cause urinary tract infection, and Serratia ficaria, which can cause respiratory infections? Getting in the habit of removing your shoes at the door will help in maintaining a healthy home.
5. Clean your cell phone. Your phone is covered in germs: 25,127 bacteria per square inch makes this device one of the dirtiest objects we come in contact with every day. And we put it up to our faces, our kitchen tables, and on public surfaces! During a pandemic scare, it would be ideal not to the take the phone out in public. If you do, you will want to clean your phone with a disinfectant every day and anytime you set it on a public surface. Preventative action stops infection.

6. Clean hands are a must. Let's be honest, kids are not very vigilant about keeping their hands clean. One tip we have done in our household is to keep hand sanitizers or hand wipes around busy areas in the home. We have a bottle of hand sanitizer near the bathroom sinks, kitchen sinks, where we keep our car keys. We have also given our kids travel hand sanitizers to put in their backpacks and sports bags.

Make Your Own Hand Sanitizer

- 1½ ounces of isopropyl alcohol
- 1 tablespoon pure aloe vera
- 15 drops essential oils (see our favorite combinations below)

Combine all ingredients in a 2-ounce plastic spray bottle and shake well to combine. Adjust scent by adding more essential oil.

Here are some of our favorite essential oil scent combinations:

- **Germ-Fighting:** If you have heard of the 4 thieves oil, then you know it has germ-fighting potential. You'll love this scent combination of 5 drops each of clove, lemon, cinnamon, eucalyptus, rosemary.
- **Calming and Preventative:** This is one of my favorites and it always calms me when I put it on. All you need is 10 drops of lavender oil, 5 drops of lemon oil.
- **Clean and Simple:** If you like the classics, you will love this scent combo. All you need is 5 drops lemon oil, 5 drops grapefruit oil and 5 drops of thyme oil.

7. Practice what you preach! We tell our kids all the time not to share food or drinks, avoid touching your eyes,

nose, and mouth until you've effectively washed your hands, and cover your mouth when coughing or sneezing. But are you guilty of some of these? I know I have been on occasion! None of us are perfect, but we need to try to set a good example for our children to follow!

8. Dust your house. As mentioned earlier, germs travel on dust particles and if kicked up in the air can cause you to breathe the dusty germs in. You should also vacuum first, then wipe any dust kicked up from the vacuum off surfaces.

9. Isolate the sick. It's such a hard thing to do, especially when it's a little kid, but anyone in the home who is sick should stay in their room away from other family members and communal areas. If they stay in a room that is well-ventilated, they are less likely to pass on the illness.

When searching out cleaning products at the store, look for products advertising anti-microbial properties. Bleach, Purell, and Lysol all make products that can kill viruses.

For disinfection, diluted household bleach solutions, alcohol solutions with at least 70% alcohol, and most common EPA-registered household disinfectants should be effective.

Diluted household bleach solutions can be used if appropriate for the surface. Follow manufacturer's instructions for application and proper ventilation. Check to ensure the product is not past its expiration date. Never mix household bleach with ammonia or any other cleanser. Unexpired household bleach will be effective against coronaviruses when properly diluted. Prepare a bleach solution by mixing:

• 5 tablespoons (1/3 cup) bleach per gallon of water or
• 4 teaspoons bleach per quart of water

If surfaces are dirty, they should be cleaned using a detergent or soap and water prior to disinfection. A trick to cleaning surfaces properly is to spray disinfecting products about 6–8 inches from surfaces and make sure the product stays on a surface for at least 10 seconds before wiping it down.

The Sick Room

To decrease the chances of an infectious illness spreading and infecting other household members, it is important that every effort be made to keep the illness in a contained area. A sick room in the home can be created and assist in limiting the number of people who have close contact with the sick person.

Characteristics of the ideal sick room

To ensure that the sickness is as contained as possible, set up the sick room in a bedroom or another separate room in the house. Poor ventilation systems have a capacity to spread droplets infected with contagious disease when someone sneezes or coughs. While those systems already use filters and other methods to scrub the air clean, some diseases have a capacity to spread through the air. Moreover, blowing cold air at night has a tendency to dry out nasal passages, thus making the body more susceptible to viruses entering through the nose while you sleep. If an airborne virus is threatening the home, close the vents to rooms so that contaminated air is not circulated through the home. Added measure for this would be to use plastic sheeting and duct tape to block the vents.

That said, a room with a window that opens can easily circulate air in the sick room. Another important characteristic of a sick room would be for the room to have an attached bathroom with a sink and running water. The less the sick person has to leave the room, the better. Further, to err on the side of caution and make sure the illness is not spread into other parts of the household, create a secured area using plastic sheeting on the outside of the room to remove clothing and items worn inside the room. A trash can could be added to discard items.

Prevention is key

To avoid other family members falling ill, limit the exposure of people coming into the sick room. This includes making sure that any communal areas (kitchen, bathroom, etc.) be thoroughly cleaned with disinfectant each day to avoid the transmission of germs. Towels, water bottles, drinking glasses, and other personal care items used by the sick person should not be used by other family members.

To further safeguard your home and the occupants inside the home, have all necessary supplies and items for the sick room present beforehand. Doing so will reduce the likelihood of contaminating other members and areas of the household andmake for easy accessibility, as well as provide a more controlled environment.

Similar to other emergencies, we simply prepare as much as we can because any steps taken toward preparedness are better than none at all. That said, due to the erratic nature of pandemics, it is vital to have all supplies ahead of time to avoid any exposure.

10 Preventative Measures for Sick Rooms

1. Line a mattress with plastic sheeting to prevent bodily fluids from soaking in.
2. All tissues, utensils, equipment, bedding, and clothing in contact with the sick person should be handled as if the germs of the illness were on them. Dishes and equipment should be washed in hot soapy water or wiped with 10% bleach or other disinfectant.
3. Use disposable dishes when possible so they can be discarded in garbage bags in the sick room.
4. Place all used tissues directly into a zip-loc plastic bag that can be closed at the top before leaving the sick room. Have alcohol-based hand cleaning solution at

the bedside so the person can wash their hands after they cough or sneeze.

5.   Gently fold or roll clothing and bedding into a plastic bag, being careful not to shake them, possibly releasing the germs into the air. Clothing and bedding should be washed in hot water. Note: Many of us are in the habit of grabbing dirty laundry and "hugging it" against our bodies. A sick person's towels, bedding, and clothes (and the clothes of the caregiver) are full of the germs that got them sick, so don't "hug" dirty clothes as you take them to the washer. This could spread the germs onto you. Transport dirty clothes in a plastic bag. Wash your hands after loading them into the washer. Wash clothing with color safe bleach and be sure you clean your washing machine with bleach to kill any lingering viruses after you've washed all the clothes.

6.   Clean items in the room with a 10% bleach solution (made by combining 1 ounce of bleach with 9 ounces of water) or other disinfectant. Clean bathroom faucets and sink with 10% bleach or disinfectant wipes after the sick person has used them.

7.   Wash your hands or use alcohol-based hand sanitizer on your hands every time you leave the room. If disposable gloves are available, they can be worn while in the room but they should be removed in the room and discarded in the room, and then your hands must be washed.

8.   Depending on how infectious the disease is, limit the people in close contact (within 6 feet) of the sick person. Keep the door to the sick room closed. Have a bell or cell phone by the bedside so the person can call for assistance when needed. If respiratory masks (N95 masks) are available, they should be worn by the sick person and the caretaker when they are in close contact.

9. Wear a disposable gown, Tyvek suit, or your personal protective equipment ensuring that you are fulling protected from contracting the contagious illness.

Cleaning and disinfecting the sick room

1. Wear PPE: wear gloves, a surgical mask in accordance with droplet precautions, or use a respirator when airborne precautions are warranted by the circumstances, and face and eye protection if cleaning within 6 feet of a coughing patient.
2. A gown must be worn when cleaning a patient infected with COVID-19 especially if soiling of the clothes or uniform has blood or other potentially infectious materials may occur.
3. Use bleach or a disinfectant when cleaning.
4. Give special attention to frequently touched surfaces (e.g., bedrails, bedside and over-bed tables, TV controls, call buttons, telephones, lavatory surfaces including safety/pull-up bars, doorknobs, commodes, and ventilator surfaces) in addition to floors and other horizontal surfaces.

Some items to consider when stocking a sick room are:

- Tyvek protective suit and shoe covers
- Plastic sheeting
- Bed with linens, pillow and blanket
- Small wastebasket or a bucket lined with a plastic garbage bag.
- Gallon-sized zip-loc bags
- Pitcher or large bottle for water
- Large plastic dishpan
- A portable toilet and human waste bags
- Vaporizer and air purifier

- Clipboard with paper and a pen for writing in the daily log.
- Clock
- Hand crank or battery-powered radio
- Good source of light
- Flashlight with extra batteries
- A clothing hamper or a garbage can lined with a plastic garbage bag can be used to collect soiled clothing and bedding items before they are washed.
- A bell or a noisemaker to call for assistance.
- Thermometer
- Tissues
- Hand wipes or a waterless hand sanitizer
- Bleach or disinfectant
- Cotton balls
- Rubbing alcohol, disinfectant, or bleach
- Measuring cup capable of holding 8 ounces or 250 ml
- Over-the-counter medications for use in the sick room
- Protective eye gear
- Protective clothing
- Disposable aprons or smocks (at least 2 cases)
- Duct tape for sealing off doorways and vents
- Latex household disposable cleaning gloves
- Disposable nitrile gloves (2-3 boxes)
- Garbage bags
- Trash can
- N95 masks or N100 respirator masks

How to Protect Yourself in a Viral Hot Zone

Here's a scenario:

A fast-moving virus has infected 6 people in your sleepy little town and no one knows for sure where the infection started. All you know is 4 of the infected live within 10 miles of you and now your 14-year-old daughter is showing symptoms.

You alert health authorities and they tell you that her symptoms are mild and that she should stay in an isolated part of the house and you need to quarantine yourself for 14 days. They stress the importance of personal protective equipment anytime you are in contact with her to protect yourself.

When we find ourselves in a viral hot zone or a loved one has come down with a pandemic illness, it is important for you to protect yourself with personal protective equipment (PPE). This is protective clothing, helmets, goggles, or other garments or equipment designed to protect the wearer's body to prevent self-contamination.

Critical PPE items include:

- Disposable Nitrile gloves (non-sterile)
- Disposable gowns
- N95 facemasks
- Goggles or disposable face shield

Read more about PPE in Chapter 4.

Personal Nonpharmaceutical Interventions (NPIs)

Your main priority during a pandemic is to limit the spread of germs and prevent infections. To do so, you must practice personal nonpharmaceutical interventions (NPIs).

Personal NPIs are everyday preventive actions, apart from pharmaceutical interventions such as getting vaccinated and taking medicine that can help keep yourself and others from getting and spreading respiratory illnesses..

During a flu pandemic there are measures you can take in addition to these everyday preventive actions. They include staying home if you have been exposed to a family or household member who is sick, covering your nose and mouth with a mask or cloth if you are sick and around people or at a mass gathering in a community where the pandemic is already occurring.

Many of these are no-brainers, but I have included a few more to consider as my Personal NPIs for times of a pandemic concern:

1. No handshaking or high fives. Use a fist bump, light bow, or elbow bump.
2. Use ONLY your knuckle to touch light switches, elevator buttons, etc. Lift the gasoline dispenser with a paper towel or use a disposable glove.
3. Do not open doors with your hand, unless there is no other way to open to the door. Use a closed fist or hip if possible. As well, avoid handrails. Touching a handrail is like shaking hands with 10,000 people. If you have to, find a place to thoroughly wash your hand or use hand sanitizer as soon as possible. Another option is to wear disposable gloves in public places.
4. If provided, use disinfectant wipes at stores. Wipe grocery carts down, especially the child seat.
5. Wash your hands with soap for 20 seconds and/or use a greater than 60% alcohol-based hand sanitizer (see recipe above) whenever you return to your car, your home, or any activity that involves locations where other people have been. Tip: if you are at a restaurant, clean your hands after touching the menu and before you eat.
6. Stop eating communal appetizers and foods like chips and dip.
7. Keep hand sanitizer with you at the entrance to your home, in the car, in the bathroom, and even in the kitchen. It's better to be safe than sorry.
8. If possible, cough or sneeze into a disposable tissue and throw away immediately. Use your elbow only if you must. The clothing on you will contain an infectious virus that can be passed on for up to a week or more.

9. Stop touching your eyes, nose, and mouth. Here's a scary fact, we touch our face over 90 times a day. During a pandemic scare, this is playing a game of Russian roulette with your immune system. We all know that we touch our faces constantly and kids do it even more. Being conscious of this and trying to avoid doing it during the flu season can cut down virus transmission significantly. If you have to, wear a disposable facemask for a week and train yourself to stop touching your face.

10. Stay away from highly trafficked areas if you can. The more people you come in contact with the greater the chance of you contracting a deadly contagion.

The 5 Ps of Preparedness for ANY Disaster or Crisis

Emergencies typically occur with little or no warning. As a result, many are caught off guard and are ill equipped to handle such a sudden crisis. Preparing ahead of time seems like the only logical way to handle this issue. However, the fact remains that a majority of our neighbors and fellow citizens are not prepared. One of the common reasons why people do not prepare is because of the overwhelming nature of it all.

Breaking up the enormity of preparedness into smaller compartmentalized sections will help you concentrate on one task at a time until the end goal is met. Follow the 5 Ps with any disaster you are planning for:

Prioritize

Decide what types of disasters you are planning for (weather related, natural disasters, biological, economic or personal disasters), and prioritize what your emergency plans will be by which emergencies are most likely to occur in your area. Also, do not limit your emergency preparedness organization to natural or economic disasters. Go a step further and plan for personal disasters that also tend to occur without warning (unemployment, divorce, death in the family).

Plan

Planning is the key to survival. Having a plan in place to help determine what steps need to be taken by you and your family members when an emergency arise will ensure that all preparedness needs are covered.

Also, having a preparedness guide to assist during the initial disaster preparation will help in determining what steps need to be taken by you and your family members when an emergency does arise. When planning for a disaster follow these protocols:

- Have a plan in place (choose the location, let family members know where your destination is, the contact information, a secondary destination, etc.).
- Decide on the duration of the disaster you are planning for (3-day, 2 week, short-term or longer-term disasters).
- Create a financial plan on how much money you can contribute to your preparedness budget.
- Keep the basic needs in mind: food, water, shelter, clothing, safety, and communication.
- Try to find items that are lightweight, functional, and versatile so that if you have to carry them for long periods it will not be a strain.
- Also, ensure that you have contingency plans put in place in case your first plan does not work out.

Prepare

Remember to prepare for disasters in a way that is financially responsible. Over time, by accumulating a few preparedness supplies each month, you will create a preparedness foundation that you can fall back on. Remember to use your lists to ensure that you are purchasing the needed items for the disaster you are preparing for. Have a well-rounded short-term supply to compliment your long-term food items. Store your emergency supplies in an easy-to-access part of your home where natural elements such as sunlight and moisture are not an issue.

Practice

The best way to be better prepared for emergencies is through knowledge and practice. Read, watch, and walk through any information on disaster preparedness you can get your hands on. We have all heard the saying, "Practice makes perfect." This is no different, in the case of preparedness. Consistent practice will turn your life-saving plans into muscle memory. This rehearse-to-be-ready concept is how many emergency personnel and even athletes train to condition their mind and body. However, being prepared is not only having supplies, it is having a skill set to fall back on if need be.

Peace of mind

The end result of the aforementioned is simply peace of mind. Knowing which disasters may affect your family and having the necessary supplies in place to handle these disruptions in our daily lives will ensure that all of your preparedness concerns are covered. Taking that extra time to prepare can make all the difference if an unexpected disaster occurs.

Critical Pandemic Supplies to Store Away

Now that you have prepared your home, it is important to prepare the supplies. Because we never know if a pandemic is going to be short-lived or longer felt, it is better to err on the side of caution and over plan when it comes to immediate needs like water and food. Both water and food will be consumed eventually whether or not the pandemic fizzles out, so it's not wasteful to overstock, but it can be perilous to under-stock. As well, consider that in the event of a fast-moving pandemic, there may be loved ones who were not able to get supplies in time, so if you're over prepared, you'll be able to share with them.

One of my favorite phrases that I tell new preppers is that "your preps are your lifeline." It is always good practice to put measures in place before a disaster is upon us in order to have these lifelines available to us when we need them the most. But sometimes time is not on our side. The CDC suggests that for this COVID-19 pandemic, a person should have a two-week preparedness supply. In this book we are suggesting a month's supply of food, water, and critical supplies.

There are multiple benefits to this: 1. Having a month of supplies means you will not be underprepared for this type of disaster or have to panic shop at the last minute. 2. You will not have to go to the store during a peak pandemic event and risk being contaminated by a communicable disease while shopping. 3. Having all your supplies in place means you will not need to be dependent on the local government for hand-outs and MREs. 4. You will have extra in case a family member needs help.

Another reason we recommend storing one month (or longer) of supplies for pandemic preparedness is, let's say that you were able to get all of your necessary supplies and prepped for the recommended two-week emergency that the CDC suggests. When those supplies dwindle, you and every other person who only prepared for two weeks will be going out and possibly reintroducing the contagious disease back into the community. If you were able to prepare for two weeks longer than everyone else, you can continue to distance yourself from the population while you observe what happens with the contagion and whether or not it will continue to spread.

Your preparedness efforts will need to concentrate on the following:

- Water

- Food
- Sanitation
- Alternative power
- Communication
- Security

(Also see Chapter 4 for recommended medical supplies.)

Water

Water is sometimes taken for granted until it isn't readily available. Two common concerns during a pandemic are waterborne pathogens and our home utilities stopping due to contagion spread.

During times of pandemics, your water may be contaminated. Some pathogens such as legionnaires disease is waterborne and has the capacity to create large outbreaks if left untreated. Other common water-borne diseases that could cause widespread epidemics are cryptosporidiosis (Cryptosporidium), Escherichia coli O157:H7 Infection (E. coli O157), and Hemolytic Uremic Syndrome (HUS), Giardiasis (Giardia), Norovirus Infection (aka Norwalk virus, calicivirus, viral gastroenteritis), Shigellosis (Shigella).

Although COVID-19 is not thought to be a water-borne virus, we should also consider what happens if our utilities crumble because utility workers stop showing up for work for fear of getting ill. The constant flow of water in the home may come to a screeching halt, and not having any stored away or a means to treat it would be deadly.

If there is fear of public spread pathogens or mandatory quarantines, local governments or utility companies may impose emergency restrictions. Although the effects of a pandemic on a workforce are unpredictable, some workers will not chance being exposed to a deadly pathogen. As well, take into consideration that smaller utility companies may be hardest hit. Thirty to 40% of a utility that has 400 or 500 employees is going to be different than 30 to 40% of a utility that has 10 employees. While most local governments will do all they can to ensure homes have electricity and water, sometimes things happen that are beyond their control and it is important to plan for it.

How much to prepare

Keep in mind that, in terms of survival, water is your most important prep. You need water for consumption, food preparation, and for sanitary needs. Ensure that you have a large quantity of water stored away for emergency use.

Emergency organizations suggest 1 gallon of drinking water per person per day for 30 days. Bear in mind this is only for drinking needs and does not take into account sanitation and food preparation. If one goes by this suggestion, to have 1 gallon per person per day, a family of 5 will need 35 gallons of water per week.

Why water bottles have expiration dates

While picking up cases of bottled water for your emergency supplies, you may notice the expiration date stamped on the bottle and wonder why.

Of course, water doesn't expire, but you should still check the expiration date on the bottle before you drink it. According to LiveScience.com, there a few different reasons why water bottles come with expiration dates, and the first one, you shouldn't worry too much about, but the second one should make you think twice.

Since water is a consumable product, regulations and laws require bottles to be stamped with an expiration date even though water doesn't ever "expire." Rational people understand this, but the government feels the need to step in and protect us from ourselves anyway.

Unlike the water itself, which has existed on Earth for 4.5 billion years, that manufactured plastic bottle only has so much time before it "goes bad." The plastic bottles that water comes packaged in (usually polyethylene terephthalate (PET) for retail bottles and high-density polyethylene (HDPE) for water cooler jugs) will eventually fail (expire) and begin to leach plastic chemicals into the water with an effect on the overall taste. So if you happen to find a water bottle well past its printed expiration date in your home, it's probably safe to drink, if you don't mind the chemical bits of bottle which have broken down and are now swirling around in it, but you should also be aware of the fact that it might not be super fresh tasting anymore either. In a life and death situation, you could drink well-expired bottled water and probably be alright. But there are many options for storing water that could help you avoid drinking the plastic.

That said, storing water for a disaster or emergency should be done in only food grade containers. You can avoid plastics such as HDPE and PET to prevent the leaching of chemicals, but those are, technically "food grade" plastics (according to the FDA, so take that with a grain of salt) and you may not have a way around it. Also, choosing BPA-free containers will be safer as well. If water is not stored correctly, it can (and will) become toxic. You can minimize the chances of plastic chemicals leaching into your water if you store it in a cool dry place. Direct sunlight will break down the plastic more quickly. But if there is any doubt in your mind at all about the integrity of your container, trust your gut over the labels and do not store water in that container even if the FDA says it is safe to do so. There are plenty of other options.

You can purchase 5-gallon water bottles at the store and store them for short-term emergencies. Another short-term water suggestion is a water containment system that fits inside your bathtub. Commonly called the WaterBOB®, it holds up to 100 gallons of fresh drinking water in any standard bathtub in the event of an emergency. Constructed of heavy duty food grade plastic, the WaterBOB® keeps water fresh and clean for drinking, cooking, washing, and flushing. This water storage method should be used when a disaster is imminent and about to hit. Note: As a backup plan, consider investing in manual water pumps, tarps, rain gutters for the home to collect rain-water and condensation from the ground, trees, and bushes. This could save your life!

Health officials may request that each household treat their water either by boiling it, chemically treating, or using a filtration system.

4 Ways to Purify Water

Below are four ways to eliminate impurities from drinking water. In addition, it would be ideal to have some tools to filter water such as a portable filtration system like a Berkey Water Filtration System or even the portable filtration system like a Katadyn water filter.

Boiling: This is, by far, the easiest and safest method of treating water. Boil the water to a rolling boil for 1 full minute, keeping in mind that some water will evaporate. Let the water cool before drinking. Here's a tip: Boiled water will taste better if you put oxygen back into it by pouring the water back and forth between two clean containers. This also will improve the taste of stored water.

Distillation involves boiling water and then collecting only the vapor that condenses. The condensed vapor will not in-clude salt or most other impurities. To distill, fill a pot halfway with water. Tie a cup to the handle on the pot's lid so that the cup will hang right-side-up when the lid is upside-down (make sure the cup is not dangling into the water) and boil the water for 20 minutes. The water that drips from the lid into the cup is distilled.

Chemical treatment of water. If boiling water is not a pos-sibility, then chemical disinfection is advised for water purity. You can do so using bleach or purification tablets.

- **Using Bleach:**

1. Filter the water using a piece of cloth or coffee filter to remove solid particles.
2. Bring it to a rolling boil for about one full minute.
3. Let it cool at least 30 minutes. Water must be cool or the chlorine treatment described below will be useless.
4. Add 16 drops of liquid chlorine bleach per gallon of water, or 8 drops per 2-liter bottle of water. Stir to mix. Sodium hypochlorite of the concentration of 5.25% to 6% should be the only active ingredient in the bleach. There should not be any added soap or fragrances. A major bleach manufacturer has also added Sodium Hydroxide as an active ingredient, which they state does not pose a health risk for water treatment. Make sure the bleach is fragrance free before it is used.
5. Let stand 30 minutes.
6. If it smells of chlorine, you can use it. If it does not smell of chlorine, add 16 more drops of chlorine bleach per gallon of water (or 8 drops per 2-liter bottle of water), let stand 30 minutes, and smell it again. If it smells of chlorine, you can use it. If it does not smell of chlorine, discard it and find another source of water.
7. To get rid of the "chlorine taste" in the water: add vitamin c tablets to the water after the purification treatment has finished. This is a good tip to keep in mind when children are drinking the water. They tend to put their noses up at water that has funny smells or tastes.

Purification Tablets: Purification tablets such as chlorine tablets, iodine tablets, and Micropur tablets can assist in removing viruses, bacteria, cryptosporidium, and Giardia in the water. Follow the instructions recommended by the manufacturer. If a person is using iodine tablets, the iodine must be stored in a dark container. Sunlight can affect the iodine's potency. Additionally, iodine has been shown to be more effective than chlorine treatment tablets. Please note that chlorine tablets can be used in lieu of iodine tablets for persons with iodine allergies. Persons with thyroid problems or on lithium, women over fifty, and pregnant women should consult their physician prior to using iodine for purification.

Tips for water supplies

Store containers in a cool, dry place away from direct sunlight. Because most plastic beverage containers degrade over time, store them away from heat and light to prevent leakage. Because hydrocarbon vapors can penetrate polyethylene plastics, store water in plastic containers away from gasoline, kerosene, pesticides, or similar substances.

1. To ensure your water supply is fresh, rotate it regularly.
2. Inspect your water supply at least every six months to see whether the containers have leaks or if any of the above problems have occurred.
3. Don't forget to have water stored for pets.
4. Look around for local water sources in your area that you can access for a back-up water supply.

Food

The timing of pandemic emergencies can be rather sudden and if you do not have supplies on hand, you may have to run to the store and brave the crowds of panicked shoppers. One way to remedy this is to have a 30-day supply of shelf-stable foods ready to go. In times of virulent outbreaks, this can save you time and sanity because you have everything you need to sustain you. While we encourage every family to prepare before an emergency or the disaster event hits the news, sometimes life gets in the way and our budgets get tight. If the panic buying ensues and people realize that they may need to begin to prepare for a possible pandemic or a widespread outbreak in their area, here are some tips to beat the lines.

1. **Shop at the local grocery stores.** If big box stores are out of stock, smaller Mom and Pop stores may still have the items you need or can give you personalized responses about when they are restocking. Also, if you are looking for paper goods like toilet paper or paper towels or disinfectant, dish soap or cleaners, consider going to your local Home Depot or Lowes store. They should have an untapped supply.
2. **Shop at night or first thing in the morning.** Shopping during times when most people are home is a great way to beat the crowds and get what you need before everyone else has a chance to show up.
3. **Order online.** Order your groceries from the convenience of your own home. No crowds, no panic. Just you clicking away! For a small fee, many stores have online buying options. If COVID19- continues to spread, this may be the new way to shop. It cuts down on social interaction and being in crowded places, keeps you away from dirty credit card machines, and helps the stores keep up with demand.
4. **Shop at the Dollar Store.** Don't underestimate what you can find at the Dollar Store!

---

30 Survival Items You Can Find at the Dollar Store

1. Paper plates and plastic utensils
2. Zip-loc storage bags
3. Water (1 gallon per day)
4. Salt and pepper
5. Spices and condiments
6. Cereal
7. Peanut butter
8. Juice per family member
9. Canned vegetables and fruit
10. Boxed dinners (macaroni and cheese, hamburger helper, etc.)

11. Cans of meat per family member (tuna, salmon, chicken, Spam, etc.)
12. Canned soup or stew
13. Non-perishable items (saltine crackers, graham crackers, oatmeal, granola bars, pasta, etc.)
14. Hand-operated can opener
15. Multi-vitamins
16. Flashlights
17. Batteries
18. Weatherproof tape
19. Trash bags
20. Soap
21. Cleaning sponges
22. Bleach
23. Toothpaste/toothbrush
24. Crisco (can use as makeshift emergency candles, fire starters, etc.)
25. First aid items such as antibiotic ointment, band-aids, gauze, elastic bandages, Tylenol
26. Toilet paper and paper towels
27. Feminine needs
28. Cigarette lighters and/or matches
29. Candles
30. Canning jars

Building an emergency pantry

Building an emergency pantry is one of those lifelines that takes both time and planning to make it fully functional. Ideally, you want to store shelf stable foods that your family normally consumes, as well as find foods that are multi-dynamic and serve many purposes.

You need to assume that electricity could go out, therefore look to foods that do not require refrigeration. Stick to classic food staples and build upon your supply each time you go to the store.

Before you begin, take inventory of what you already have. Chances are, you already have the beginnings of a solid emergency food pantry. While you are doing an inventory of your food and supplies, make a list of items you need to restock or purchase.

A few other points to consider when starting an emergency food pantry are:

- Store emergency foods that will not require refrigeration and should require little electricity or fuel to prepare.
- The food should have a long shelf life.
- It should provide ample nutrition and contain little salt.

The following foods are all popular food staples that should be considered "must-haves" for your emergency pantries. The advantages to storing these items is that they encompass all the key consideration points listed above. Best of all, these items are very affordable and versatile, thus making them worthy of being on your storage shelves for extended emergencies.

Top 25 Survival Foods to Store in Your Emergency Pantry

This list is based on the suggested items outlined in *The Prepper's Cookbook*. Stock up on the following items today to get your prepper pantry ready for the next extended emergency:

1. Canned fruits, vegetables, meats, and soups
2. Dried legumes (beans, lentils, peas)
3. Crackers
4. Nuts
5. Pasta sauce
6. Peanut butter

7. Pasta
8. Flour (white, whole wheat)
9. Seasonings (vanilla, salt, pepper, paprika, cinnamon, pepper, taco seasoning, etc.)
10. Sugar
11. Bouillon cubes or granules (chicken, vegetable, beef)
12. Kitchen staples (baking soda, baking powder, yeast, vinegar)
13. Honey
14. Unsweetened cocoa powder
15. Jell-O or pudding mixes
16. Whole grains (barley, bulgur, cornmeal, couscous, oats, quinoa, rice, wheat berries)
17. Nonfat dried milk
18. Plant-based oil (corn oil, vegetable oil, coconut oil, olive oil)
19. Cereals
20. Seeds for eating and sprouting
21. Popcorn (not the microwavable kind)
22. Instant potato flakes
23. Packaged meals (macaroni and cheese, hamburger helper, Ramen noodles, etc.)
24. Purified drinking water
25. Fruit juices, teas, coffee, drink mixes

How to build a pantry stocked with nutritious, energizing foods

The foods you store for emergencies should provide you with the energy you need during challenging times. Finding foods that are high in complex carbs and dietary fiber are more efficient from a dietary standpoint and will keep you feeling fuller longer.

When selecting foods to add to your emergency pantry, focus on the most nutrient-dense items you can find that are also shelf-stable, with a focus on macronutrients. Macronutrients are compounds found in all foods that humans consume in the largest quantities, providing the bulk of our calories (energy) from our diets. The three main categories are protein, carbohydrate, and fat.

Protein: Protein is made up of amino acids, which are the building blocks for our bodies. If we consume excess protein in our diets, our bodies will usually find a way to use it; we don't store a lot of extra amino acids like we do carbohydrates and fat. Because we either use or excrete extra protein, we need to replenish it through our diets.

Protein sources include eggs, poultry, meat, protein bars, protein powder, jerky or air-dried beef, dehydrated meat, bone broth, protein pancakes or waffles, beans or lentils, dried milk.

Carbohydrates: These energy powerhouses come in second to protein, and fat takes third place.

- Whole grain, rice, granola and dry cereals, quinoa, wheat, faro, etc.
- Dehydrated fruits and vegetables
- Freeze-dried fruits and vegetables: Freeze-dried foods are emergency pantry favorites because their shelf life is much longer compared to dehydrated foods. Due to the freeze-drying process, freeze-dried foods are more expensive, but can last 25 years or longer. So, if you're looking to ensure your long-term food needs are met, this is a good investment.
- Leafy greens and sprouts have healthy carbohydrates, so do not forget those! Many preppers find solace in growing produce from their gardens and preserving the fresh grown fruits and vegetables. Doing so gives them a constant supply of food to put away and seeds for the next year (provided that the seeds they use are non-GMO).

Fiber is also filling, so including it in meals can reduce mindless snacking (which humans are prone to do when emotionally eating or if boredom sets in—and let's face it, being stuck indoors for days on end can get boring).

- Fruits such as bananas, oranges, apples, mangoes, strawberries, raspberries.
- Vegetables that are darker in color have the higher the fiber content.
- Beans and legumes are flavorful, fiber-filled additions to salads, soups, and chilis.
- Breads and grains like whole grains, wheat berries, rice, faro, oats, etc.

Fat sources that are solid at room temperature last longer on your pantry shelf. Fat sources can go rancid over time, and not only do they taste terrible when that happens, but they also aren't good for your health. To increase the life of your fat sources, store them in a cool dark place, out of direct sunlight. Don't let water get into the containers and use a clean utensil every time you scoop a bit out.

- Ghee, coconut oil, olive oil, nuts and seeds, nut butters.

Beverages: Of course, water should be your top priority when it comes to building your emergency pantry. However, there are various reasons you may want to include other things to drink in your emergency pantry. Many of us can't imagine going a day without coffee, for example. In fact, during a long emergency situation—especially during the colder months—coffee can be a great source of comfort. Thankfully, there are ways to prepare coffee without electricity, should your power go out.

- Instant coffee, powdered milk, rice milk, almond milk, and other non-dairy beverages can be stored in the pantry until ready to use (must be kept cold after opening, so buy small containers if you won't use them up in one day).

- Tea can provide comfort and nutrients during emergency situations, so consider keeping a variety of herbal options in your pantry.
- Flavored drink powders like Tang can also be a nice change and provide some valuable nutrition.

When the grocery stores go empty, these four tips can keep you alive

The first food items that will sell out mostly consist of things that are already cooked or prepared in some way, including canned foods, frozen dishes, and bread. Fresh meat and eggs also disappear fast.

1. Instead of bread, go straight for the flour. Don't worry if you can't find any yeast. You can always make hardtack, tortillas, or naan. You might also find that the sacks of dried rice and beans won't disappear until after the canned foods go. When combined, these two make a complete protein and are perfect for emergency food meals. Keep cooking times in mind with the beans and go for small beans like navy or lentils.

2. If you find that the produce section is stripped bare, go to the supplement aisle instead. There you'll find all of the vitamins and minerals that are normally found in fresh produce. Look for food based or whole food vitamins. You'll also find protein powders that can at least partially substitute fresh meat. As well, look for seeds to sprout. Sprouts provide the highest amount of vitamins, minerals, proteins, and enzymes of any food per unit of calorie. Enzymes are essential because they heal the body, cleanse the body, prevent diseases, enhance the overall functioning of bodily organs, aid in digestion, and removes gas from the stomach. If there are no vitamins, head over to the garden center for non-gmo seeds.

3. And finally, instead of trying to find butter, which will be one of the first food items to disappear, try looking for alternatives. Remember, you need fats in your diet. Healthy oils like coconut oil or avocado oil provide nutrition and can be used for cooking and added to coffee, oats, beverages, and other foods. In addition, granola and nuts are great to have on hand. Nuts are calorie dense and full of fiber to help you stay full longer. Due to the high protein count of this natural food, it can be an efficient meat replacement too. Look for non-salted nut varieties to keep you hydrated longer. Nuts are packed with calories and can go without refrigeration for weeks without spoiling. Alternatively, if all the healthy oils and nuts have been taken, look for some lard. It's sometimes labeled "manteca." It will probably be overlooked, but has just as many calories as butter, and lasts a long time.

Foods to manage stress

At best, stress can interfere with your happiness and productivity.

At worst, stress can be a slow killer: It can adversely affect your immune, cardiovascular, neuroendocrine, and central nervous systems, especially when it is experienced chronically.

Fortunately, there is a way to naturally manage that. This is one of the many reasons we promote eating a nutrient dense diet in times of emergencies.

- **Folate (also known as Vitamin B9):** Helps your body produce mood-regulating neurotransmitters, including serotonin and dopamine. Folate is crucial for proper brain function and plays an important role in mental and emotional health. Studies show that folate paired with B12 can help treat depression. Dietary sources: dark leafy greens, asparagus, turnips, beets, Brussels sprouts, beans, avocado, milk

- **Vitamin B1 (thiamine):** Sometimes called an "anti-stress" vitamin, B1 can help strengthen the immune system and improve the body's ability to withstand stressful conditions. Dietary sources: pork, beef, poultry, legumes, black beans, seeds, nuts.
- **Vitamin B2 (riboflavin):** Studies have shown B2 can help support adrenal function, help calm and maintain a healthy nervous system, and prevent or alleviate depression. Dietary sources: dairy products (like milk, cheese, and yogurt), eggs, enriched or fortified cereals and grains, meats, liver, dark greens (including asparagus, broccoli, spinach, and turnip greens), fish, poultry, and buckwheat
- **Vitamin B3 (niacin):** Mild deficiency has been associated with depression. Dietary sources: beets, brewer's yeast, salmon, swordfish, tuna, sunflower seeds, peanuts
- **Vitamin B6 (pyridoxine): helps the body make several neurotransmitters:** chemicals that carry signals from one nerve cell to another. It is needed for normal brain development and function, and helps the body make the hormones serotonin and norepinephrine, which influence mood, and melatonin, which helps regulate the body's internal "clock." Dietary sources: fortified cereal, chicken, turkey, tuna, salmon, shrimp, milk, cheese, lentils, beans, hummus (chickpeas), spinach, carrots, brown rice, sunflower seeds, bananas.
- **Vitamin B12 (cobalamin):** aids in the creation of red blood cells and nerves. Low levels of B12 can cause short-term fatigue, slowed reasoning, and paranoia, and are associated with depression. Dietary sources: fish, lean meat, poultry, eggs, milk, Swiss cheese, and fortified breakfast cereals
- **Tryptophan:** An essential amino acid (this means your body cannot produce it—you must get it from your diet), tryptophan helps your body make niacin, mel-

atonin, and serotonin. In order for tryptophan to be converted into niacin, however, your body needs to have enough iron, vitamin B 6, and vitamin B 2. Dietary sources: chicken, turkey, eggs, cheese, lentils, fish, peanuts, pumpkin and sesame seeds, milk, turkey, tofu and soy, chocolate.

- **Foods that support gut health:** Your gut loves fermented foods like yogurt (not the sugary kind), kimchi, pickles, kombucha, kefir, and sauerkraut.
- **Omega-3 fatty acids:** Omega-3 is an essential fatty acid that is important for brain health (it contributes up to 18 percent of the brain's weight!). The body does not naturally produce omega-3, so you need to get it from dietary or supplemental sources. Deficiency symptoms include fatigue, mood swings, memory decline, and depression. Dietary sources: wild-caught Alaskan salmon, sardines, anchovies, halibut, mackerel, chia seeds, flaxseeds, pumpkin seeds, walnuts, fortified foods (check labels), high-quality krill oil supplements.
- **Blueberries:** Anthocyanins, the pigments that are responsible for the deep colors of the tiny fruit, help with the brain's production of dopamine.
- **Bananas:** In order to make dopamine, your body needs the amino acid tyrosine, and bananas are a great source (almonds, avocados, eggs, beans, fish, and chicken are also decent sources). Bananas also contain B vitamins and magnesium, which can calm you down.
- **Pistachios:** One study found eating two servings of pistachios a day lowered vascular constriction during stress, which means the load on your heart is reduced since your arteries are more dilated. Choose fresh organic pistachios: conventional ones carry a high risk of contamination by a carcinogenic mold called aflatoxin, and may be bleached or fumigated during processing.

- **Oatmeal:** A complex carbohydrate, oatmeal causes your brain to produce serotonin, which creates a soothing feeling that can help you ease stress.
- **Zinc:** An essential mineral that may help reduce anxiety, zinc is found in nearly every cell of the body and plays an important role in immune system functioning. Low levels of zinc in the diet can lead to a variety of ailments, including loss of appetite, mental lethargy, and depression. Dietary sources: roasted pumpkin seeds, cashews, pine nuts, almonds, dark chocolate, cheese, oatmeal, beef, oysters, pork.
- **Vitamin C:** Studies suggest this vitamin can curb levels of stress hormones while strengthening the immune system. In one of the people with high blood pressure, blood pressure and levels of cortisol returned to normal more quickly when people took vitamin C before a stressful task. Dietary sources: cantaloupe, citrus fruits (including oranges, lemons, and grapefruit), Kiwi fruit, mango, papaya, pineapple, strawberries, raspberries, blueberries, blackberries, cranberries, watermelon, Acerola cherries, rose hips, blackcurrants, broccoli, Brussels sprouts, cauliflower, green and red peppers, spinach, cabbage, kale, turnip greens, and other leafy greens, sweet and white potatoes, tomatoes and tomato juice, winter squash.
- **Vitamin D:** Often called "the sunshine vitamin," vitamin D is unique in that it is a vitamin AND a hormone your body can make with help from the sun. But despite the ability to get vitamin D from food and the sun, an estimated 40%-75% of people are deficient. Research suggests that low levels of vitamin D are associated with mood disorders and depression. Dietary sources: salmon, tuna, mackerel, eggs, cheese, fortified foods like orange juice and milk. Some vitamin D researchers have found that somewhere between 5–30 minutes of sun exposure between 10 AM and 3 PM at least twice a

week to the face, arms, legs, or back without sunscreen usually leads to sufficient vitamin D synthesis. Indoor light therapy can help, too.

- **Chromium:** A trace mineral found in small amounts in the body, chromium plays an important role in increasing the brain's levels of serotonin, norepinephrine, and melatonin, which help regulate emotion and mood. Because chromium works directly with the brain's mood regulators, it's been found to be an effective treatment for depression. Dietary sources: broccoli, grape juice, potatoes, garlic, basil, orange juice, turkey breast, apples, bananas, green beans

- **Magnesium:** Studies found that this mineral helps ward off depression and migraines. It has also been found to function in a similar manner to lithium, which is often prescribed for bipolar disorder as a mood stabilizer. Dietary sources: almonds, hazelnuts, cashews, pumpkin seeds (1/2 cup provides almost 100% of your daily requirement), sunflower seeds, Brazil nuts, pine nuts, flaxseed, pecans, dark chocolate, bananas, strawberries, blackberries, grapefruit, figs, yogurt

- **Dark chocolate:** Chocolate is one of the most-craved foods in the world, and the reasons go beyond its pleasing taste and texture—it contains over 300 naturally-occurring chemicals, some of which make you feel happy via the release of certain neurotransmitters. Feel-good chemicals in chocolate include:
  - **Tryptophan and serotonin:** Creates feelings of relaxation and well-being
  - **Caffeine:** Psychoactive substance that creates temporary alertness
  - **Xanthines:** Mild stimulant that occurs naturally in the brain and, like caffeine, increases wakefulness
  - **Theobromine:** Stimulant and vasodilator that increases blood flow

- **Phenylethylamine:** Compound that stimulates the brain to release dopamine, a neurotransmitter associated with feelings of pleasure and motivation
- **Anandamide:** Neurotransmitter that activates pleasure receptors in the brain
- **Flavonols:** Compounds that boost blood flow to key areas of the brain for two to three hours after being metabolized. Creates effects similar to those of a mild analgesic (painkiller) like aspirin

Is freeze-dried food worth the investment?

Preppers often gravitate toward freeze-dried foods. For years, the freeze-dried food industry has profited heavily on families wanting to get their pantries emergency ready. But is it worth all the hype and money?

There are many who wonder if the investment into this long-term food source is the right one for them and have asked questions like: Can you really survive the apocalypse with freeze-dried food? How long is the shelf-life when the #10 can is opened? Are these foods nutritionally complete? What other options are there for long-term food storage?

The Pros

There are many pros to having #10 cans of this long-term food source in your prepper pantry. Freeze-dried food is flash frozen and then put in a vacuum container causing the water to vaporize and leaving the food item with 98% of its water removed. Nutritionally speaking, the food retains all the nutrients that it had in its original form after the freeze-drying process and contains little to no additives. This process keeps a majority of the nutrition intact. Gary Stoner, Ph.D., and the American Institute for Cancer Research have found that the antioxidant phytochemicals found in fresh fruits is about the same as in their freeze-dried versions. However, some ascorbic acid levels and the amount of polyphenol, a cell-protecting chemical in berries, were measurably reduced by freeze drying.

As well, the cook times are drastically reduced which is helpful during emergencies when energy must be conserved. Moreover, many find that when they are in the midst of an emergency, stress loads increase because of drastic changes and having these "just add water" meals ready to go cuts down on the stress of food preparation. It is estimated that 98% of moisture from the food is eliminated, thus reducing the weight of the food by 80%. Those who plan on evacuating will appreciate the lighter weight during transport—especially with all the other supplies they will have in their pack. Last but not least, the 25 year storage life makes this ideal for preppers who are looking for long-lasting food options. On a personal note, my family purchased freeze-dried food in 2004 and it's still just as fresh as when we opened up the first can. Keep in mind, once your freeze-dried food can is opened, the shelf life quickly diminishes and you will need to throw it out in six months, and if you live in a humid area, the shelf life could be cut in half.

The Cons
While the pros are great, it comes with a hefty price tag. You are paying for all of the specialized equipment and energy it takes to preserve the food for a long shelf life. One case of freeze-dried meals can set you back over a hundred dollars with shipping included. As well, having this type of food source for your long-term food needs will require extra space to store the food. An entire year's supply fits into a 2 ft x 3 ft area, stacked 5 ft high. As well, food cans could be strategically hidden in the home, underneath beds, above kitchen cabinets and in the closet.

If you are going back and forth about whether or not to invest in freeze-dried food or dehydrated food, here's a good answer. Because 98% of the water is removed from freeze-dried foods, it will take more water to reconstitute it for meals as opposed to dehydrated foods, which only need a fraction of the water.

Also, keep in mind that many of the freeze-dried meals are high in sodium. Many outdoor enthusiasts and hikers complain that you have to drink so much water to overcome the thirst the meals create. Make sure you have extra water on hand if you plan on using this as your main food source. As well, the high sodium can cause your bowels to become sluggish. To remedy this, purchase some over the counter meds for constipation or look for low-sodium freeze-dried options. Also consider balancing your freeze-dried meals. For example, for breakfast, eat oatmeal or granola and then have freeze-dried meat and vegetables for dinner. This will control the amount of sodium you are putting in your body.

In that same vein, I highly recommend you also invest in sprouting seeds to ensure you are getting some fresh vitamins into your daily diet.

How Much Freeze-Dried Food Do You Need?

In an emergency situation, your caloric intake will increase due to higher activity levels, thus you will be consuming more. Keep this in mind when determining what your caloric needs will be. Once you know that magic caloric number, you can begin to find out how many freeze-dried meals you need.

Can You Survive Solely on Freeze-Dried Food?

So, the question is can you survive a crisis with freeze-dried food? Yes, you can, but the real question is do you want to?

While there are pros and cons to investing in this long-term food source, above all, you are investing in food freedom and the livelihood of your family or group. My preference is to have a little bit of everything and believe in having a layered approach to emergency food sources. We plan on using our supply of freeze-dried food after we finish our perishable foods. During the time we are using up this portion of our emergency food, we plan on getting fresh food sources established.

Ultimately, when people set out on the path to prepared-ness, they turn to freeze-dried foods for a fast approach. Af-ter all, it is the healthiest and longest lasting emergency food source. Based on the price alone, it is difficult for many of us to use this as a sole emergency food source. There are less costly food storage options such as using a dehydrator to dry out food and is completely customizable to your dietary needs. As well, the further a person journeys into preparedness, the more they want to attain total self-sufficiency and look for ways to grow their own food sources through gardening and livestock.

Keep your budgets in mind before you decide to purchase bulk emergency food. You don't want to go broke getting a food pantry set up. Prep for emergencies with the layered approach mentioned above, keep your options open, and keep research-ing better ways to get your family ready for life's uncertainties.

What about dehydrated foods?

For centuries, dehydrating food has been used as a means of survival. Many consider this to be the most affordable pres-ervation method, and the best way to preserve the flavors of foods. Dehydrating vegetables and fruits for long-term storage is a great way to get needed nutrition into diets with minimal investment. The dehydration process removes moisture from the food so that bacteria, yeast, and mold cannot grow. The added benefit is the dehydration process minimally effects the nutritional content of food. In fact, when using an in-home dehydration unit, 3%–c 5% of the nutritional content is lost compared to the canning method which looses 60%–80% of the nutritional content. Additionally, vitamins A and C, carbo-hydrates, fiber, potassium, magnesium, selenium, and sodium are not altered or lost in the drying process. Therefore, the end result is nutrient packed food that can be stored long term.

Pros
Of course, the greatest aspect of this food storage method is anyone can do it. You set it and forget it! Dehydrating food

can be a way to circumvent the costliness of large quantities of already-preserved food, while complimenting your existing preparedness pantry at the same time. Not to mention, due to the drying process, dehydrated foods condense in their size thus creating a more efficient use of storage space.

Dehydrated foods are the original just add water meal! Think of the possibilities—don't limit yourself to only dehydrating your surplus vegetables and fruits. You can dehydrate meals, soups, meat, and cooked grains. They can then be combined together to create a delicious, nutritious, life-saving meal. Moreover, pre-cooking and then dehydrating your beans, grains, and pastas and then rehydrating them will drastically cut down on fuel usage during emergencies. You can dehydrate pasta meals and have them on hand for quick meals or to add to backpacks. All one needs to rehydrate their meal is to add boiling water and cover with a lid for 20–30 minutes to expedite the process.

Home dehydration has one more bonus: unlike the purchased dehydrated foods, it's not loaded with sodium unless you choose to do so.This is great if anyone in your group suffers from high blood pressure or a heart condition. It is recommended to add salt after the re-hydration process has been completed.

Cons

Keep in mind that the drawback to this food preservation method is that you will need a large amount of water in order to rehydrate the dried food. Depending on the situation, that could be a problem in an emergency. Further, when rehydrated, some foods will not take on their original shape and form. The long drying times could also pose a challenge if you plan on dehydrating large quantities of food.

5 Delicious Meal-in-a-Jar Recipes

Instant Oatmeal Mix

Makes 14 servings (1/2 cup each)

- 6 cups quick-cooking oats
- 1/3 cup dry powdered milk
- 1/4 cup powdered sugar
- 1/4 cup packed brown sugar
- 3 teaspoons ground cinnamon
- 1 teaspoon salt
- 1 cup dried fruit or nuts

1. In a large bowl, combine all of the above ingredients. Then store in airtight container in a cool dry place for up to 1 month.
2. To prepare oatmeal: Place 1/2 cup of mix and add 1/2 cup boiling water or milk to the mix and stir until oats are softened, about 2–3 minutes.

Instant Potato Flakes

Makes 1-pint jar

- 5 potatoes, peeled and chopped
- Water

1. Cover potatoes with just enough water to cover them. Over medium heat, boil potatoes for 10–15 minutes, or until soft.
2. Once potatoes are soft, drain water and mash potatoes until smooth. Do not add any milk or seasonings.
3. Set potatoes on dehydrator fruit roll sheets or a parchment paper lined dehydrator tray. Dehydrate on 145°Ffor 6 hours or until dry and all moisture is removed.

4. Break the sheets into chunks, put in the blender, and pulse until ground into flakes. The finer the flake, the stickier the potatoes will be when you reconstitute them.
5. Add to a glass jar or container and store in a cool, dry area for up to 6 months.
6. To flavor soups, casseroles, and dishes add by the tablespoon until desired thickness is met.

For Mashed Potatoes:

Add potato flakes to boiling water, then remove from heat. Add additional ingredients such as cold milk, butter, salt, and seasonings and stir in reconstituted potato flakes.

2 servings:

2/3 cup water, 1/4 teaspoon salt, 1 tablespoon butter, 1/4 cup milk, 2/3 cup flakes

4 servings:

1 1/3 cups water, 1/2 teaspoon salt, 2 tablespoons butter, 1/2 cup milk, 1 1/3 cup flakes

8 servings:

2 2/3 cups water, 1 teaspoon salt, 4 tablespoons butter, 1 cup milk, 2 2/3 cup flakes

16 servings:

5 1/3 cups water, 2 teaspoons salt, 8 tablespoons butter, 2 cups milk, 5 1/3 cups flakes

---

Instant Potato Gnocchi

Makes 4 servings

- 1 cup mashed potato flakes
- 1 cup boiling water
- 1 eggs, lightly beaten
- 1½ cups organic unbleached flour
- 1 teaspoon garlic powder
- 1 tablespoon Italian herb seasoning

- 1/4 teaspoon salt
- Water for boiling
- Pasta sauce of your choice
- Grated Parmesan cheese, optional

1. In a large bowl, add potato flakes and stir in boiling water.
2. Add egg, flour, and seasonings. On a lightly floured surface, knead for a few minutes until a soft dough forms. Divide dough into four portions.
3. On a floured surface, roll each portion into 1/2-in.-thick ropes; cut into 3/4-in. pieces. Press and roll each piece with a lightly floured fork.
4. In a large saucepan, bring water to a boil. Cook gnocchi in batches for 30–60 seconds or until they float. Remove with a slotted spoon.
5. Serve with sauce and sprinkle with cheese if desired.

Split Pea Soup

- 1 (2.75 ounce) package country gravy mix (regular or no-fat)
- 1 tablespoon chicken bouillon granules
- 2 tablespoons imitation bacon bits
- 2 teaspoons. dried celery flakes
- 2 teaspoons dried minced onion
- 1 teaspoon dried parsley flakes
- 1¼ cups dried split green peas
- 1 bay leaf

1. Mix all the ingredients in a bag and store until needed.
2. Empty 1 cup of contents for each serving into large saucepan or Dutch oven.
3. Add 1 cup water for each serving; heat to boiling, stirring often.

4. Reduce heat; cover and simmer for 1 to 1 1/2 hours or until peas are tender, stirring frequently to prevent peas from sticking.
5. Remove bay leaf.
6. Serve soup.

Shepherd's Pie

- 1 package Knorr Cream of Vegetable Soup
- 1 package chicken gravy mix
- 1/2 cup milk powder
- 3/4 cup mixed dried veggies (potatoes, carrots, peas, onions)
- 1/2 cup beef jerky, venison jerky, chicken jerky, or dehydrated ground beef (you can also use freeze-dried beef crumbles)
- 1/2 cup or more instant mashed potatoes

1. Mix everything but the potatoes in a bag.
2. Place potatoes in a second bag. Store until needed.
3. To prepare, bring 4 cups of water to boil.
4. Add everything but instant mashed potatoes.
5. Simmer 7–8 minutes.
6. Add instant mashed potatoes, cook for 1 minute, stirring constantly.
7. Remove from heat, let sit for minute.

Herbal teas

Studies have shown that sipping a few cups of tea daily reduces stress, balances health, promotes sleep, and boosts mood. Amino acids present in green and black teas have a calming effect on the body, reducing the adverse effects that stress can have.

Herbal teas date back thousands of years to ancient Egypt and China, where they would drink teas for their health promoting abilities. Egyptians, especially, would mix their tea with medications—to help the medicine go down. In ancient China, tea was discovered by happenstance when some wild leaves flew into a pot of boiling water held by Emperor Shen Nung. Legend has it that he enjoyed the smell, took a sip, and described a warm feeling, "as if the liquid was investigating every part of his body."

Now, Eastern wisdom has taught the world of the health-promoting benefits teas have to assist in body functions, prevent chronic diseases before they become problematic, and combat ailments such as high blood pressure and diabetes. Other common health benefits from drinking herbal tea include relaxation, anti-aging properties, pain reduction, weight loss, improvement in complexion, and the improvement of body systems (such as the digestive and immune system). It's no wonder so many are turning to herbal tea infusions as a natural health booster.

Tea is the ultimate health drink and fights chronic diseases. If you're looking for an all-around health drink, look no further than herbal tea.

- The antioxidants and vitamins found in herbal teas are great for helping fight disease and infections. They can protect against oxidative stress and lower the risk of chronic disease. Herbal teas in particular has the ability to boost the immune system, improve digestion, fight off colds, reduce inflammation, and lower blood pressure.

- **Herbal teas naturally clean and protect teeth.** Infused herbal teas are a way to promote good dental health as it does not erode tooth enamel. A mouth rinse can be made by preparing an herbal infused tea in the usual way, or by simply stirring herb powder into water. Hold the rinse in the mouth for a few seconds or up to several minutes, gargle, and spit out. A holistic mouth wash can be made of the following herbs: cloves, cinnamon, peppermint, or echinacea. Brew a strong tea and place it in the refrigerator for up to a week and use as a mouthwash.

- **Tea flavorfully hydrates the body.** The warm water helps the body absorb the phytonutrients and healing abilities while providing hydration to the body. Because of the high presence of antioxidants in herbal teas, it works to eliminate free radicals throughout the body and prevent oxidative stress. Some even believe that drinking tea is better for you than drinking water. Water is essentially replacing fluid. Tea replaces fluids and contains antioxidants, so it's got two things going for it.
- **Tea is beneficial for your digestive system because it can absorb gas, improve blood flow to the entire digestive tract, and eliminate free radicals that can cause an upset stomach and indigestion.** Herbal teas have phenols that can strengthen both stomach muscles and the muscles in your esophagus, which can reduce acid reflux and heartburn symptoms. Teas also enable your digestive tract to more easily absorb nutrients.
- **Relax and unwind.** There's a psychology to drinking to tea where people often feel its relaxing properties. As one article explains, the combination of warmth, aroma, and health properties boost mental and physical states of the body.

Tea has been around for generations and many of us are starting to see the ways it enhances our lives. If there is an improvement you want to make for your health, there is undoubtedly a tea to help.

Sanitation

In a pandemic, everyone will fear going to their jobs and all forms of normal life will be on hold. This includes your trash pickups. Have a basic sanitation kit and prepare for the fact that toilets may not flush and trash will not be collected.

When sanitary conditions are not up to par, there is an increase in diseases such as cholera, typhoid, and diphtheria. Typically, women and children are the most affected by poor sanitary conditions. A woman's personal hygiene is essential to her health and should be considered a priority in your sanitation preparedness measures. Taking proper precautions and stocking up on sanitary items will help eliminate most issues regarding poor sanitation.

Having a sanitation kit that is ready in times of disaster is essential to keeping your family and neighbors healthy. These kits can fit comfortably into a bucket, are affordable, and will not take up much space. Additionally, being educated on how to properly dispose of waste is a key factor in keeping everyone healthy during a disaster.

Here is what a basic sanitation kit for the home looks like:

- Disposable bucket or luggable loo
- Toilet paper (2 rolls per person/ per week)
- Rubber gloves
- Garbage bags with twist ties (for liners of toilets or for luggable loo)
- Disinfectant or bleach
- Baby wipes
- Baking soda (to help eliminate odors)
- Vinegar
- Shovel
- Women's hygiene products

In an emergency environment where the toilets stop flushing, it is essential that you know how to properly dispose of waste in order to prevent disease.

In a short-term emergency situation:

If water services are interrupted, an easy way to utilize the toilet and keep it clean is to:

- Clean and empty the water of the toilet bowl out.
- Line the bowl with a heavy-duty plastic bag.
- Once the bag has waste inside, add a small amount of deodorant such as cat litter or baking soda, as well as disinfectant, and securely tie the bag for disposal.
- A large plastic trash can (lined with a heavy-duty bag) can be used to store the bags of waste.
- Once trash services begin, the city will come and collect these.

If a portable camp toilet is used, the above mentioned can also be used. However, if the trash crews are not coming in a given amount of time, the bag of waste will need to be buried (see the proper way to bury waste below).

Officials say to avoid burying your waste, but sometimes it is necessary. However, if waste is not properly taken care of, pollution of water sources will lead to illness and disease. It also attracts flies and insects, which may spread disease further. Understand that buried feces take up to a year to decompose. Therefore, finding the right spot to bury your feces is crucial. There are biodegradable bags that a person can put their waste into. These can usually be found in the camping department of outdoor stores, or on the Internet. The bags assist the waste in decomposing faster and assist in preventing the waste from hitting major water sources. If a person does not have one of these handy bags available, the feces should be buried in "catholes" far away from water sources, campsites, and communal spot where there are a lot of humans.

- Select a cathole site far from water sources—200 feet (approximately 70 adult paces) is the recommended range.

- Select an inconspicuous site untraveled by people. Examples of cathole sites include thick undergrowth, near downed timber, or on gentle hillsides.
- If camping with a group or if camping in the same place for more than one night, disperse the catholes over a wide area; don't go to the same place twice.
- Try to find a site with deep organic soil. This organic material contains organisms which will help decompose the feces (organic soil is usually dark and rich in color.)
- If possible, locate our cathole where it will receive maximum sunlight. The heat from the sun will aid the decomposition.
- Choose an elevated site where water would not normally run off during rainstorms. The idea here is to keep the feces out of water. Over time, the decomposing feces will percolate into the soil before reaching water sources.

Disposal of feminine napkins

It is important to properly dispose of sanitary napkins, as they contain bodily fluid that could pose a health hazard to others. Methods of disposal may differ according to where you are and what you have available. However, tampons and feminine napkins do not decompose quickly. Therefore, the best way to dispose of used feminine napkins and tampons is to burn them. The fire must be very hot in order to thoroughly destroy the used items.

What if you run out of toilet paper?

This is when the you-know-what hits the fan! Fights have broken out in stores over toilet paper. In the case of an extended emergency, you may have to face the fact that you might run out of the tp. Finding toilet paper alternatives can make all the difference in this case. Mind you, these will probably not flush, so you will have to use the directions for throwing these away in a bag and either storing them for future trash disposal or burning them in the trash heap.

Toilet paper alternatives include non-poisonous leaves (mullein is great), phone books, unused coffee filters, dilapidated kitchen towels (no longer used for cleaning), restaurant napkins, bed linen strips, mail order catalogs.

Alternative Power

Disasters of any kind cause grid-down scenarios. In this case, if a pandemic ensues, people are not going to risk exposing themselves to a deadly contagion just so the public has their electricity. They want to stay home with their families too.

Prepare to live in an off-grid environment and invest in alternative means of power including rechargeable batteries, solar battery chargers, generators, ample supplies of fuel, and even a siphon for fuel. As well, if cold weather threatens the area where you live, have ample firewood and matches or a way to start a fire.

Communication

You can't cut yourself off from the world, especially in a disaster. Our normal forms of communication—television, cell phones, landlines—may not be available following a disaster. During a pandemic event, no one will want to chance being subjected to a deadly pathogen, not even to give you the 5 o'clock news. In a worse case scenario, the only messages you would be receiving are the emergency recordings on repeat.

Having alternative forms of communication like a ham radio and police scanners will be essential in having an understanding on a local, state, and federal level of what is happening. Further, having a set or two of walkie talkies to communicate with neighbors will help you safeguard your home or neighborhood.

CHAPTER 6

A Prepared Community

The resilience of our communities is solely dependent on how prepared each of their members are. A prepared populace can prevent, protect against, mitigate the effects of, respond to, and assist in the recovery from threats that pose the greatest risk.

To achieve this, our efforts must lie in readying communities and making necessary changes to control the spread of a deadly pandemic. As discussed in the previous chapter, before any of this can happen, you must ensure that your own home is adequately prepared before branching out into preparing an entire community. That said, when spikes in contagious illnesses occur in a worldwide context, community-led mitigation strategies will be implemented in order to control the virus or slow its spread through containment measures such as quarantines and travel restrictions.

Pre-Pandemic Planning

We are all aware of the strength in numbers adage. Explaining this notion can help sell the idea of a community-wide preparedness task. The odds of survival rest partly in those who we can wholeheartedly rely on. Having a large group of prepared individuals will help the general public thrive for longer increments of time because each home has the supplies and skills it needs to keep going. Moreover, communities should provide skills training to help the general public learn critical survival skills for long-term survival. Individuals bringing a variety of skills binds the group further to create a solid, well-functioning team. Along those lines, a large group of preppers can diversify themselves through cross-training in various skills.

When pandemic fears are present, local governments, businesses, and schools will be encouraged to develop plans like canceling mass gatherings or switching to teleworking.

It is important to stay informed by local government and contact them during an outbreak to find out how they are planning. Some questions to ask community leaders and emergency organizations are:

- Should the public become involved in the response? If so, in what way(s)?
- What geographical area(s) in our community has been or may be adversely impacted if a disaster occurs?
- How many people could be threatened, affected, exposed, injured, or killed?
- How will the community help elderly or disabled persons, if needed?
- Have critical infrastructures have been affected (e.g., electrical power, water)?
- In what ways can the community continue to thrive? Should the public stock up on necessary items like supplies, sanitation, telecommunications, transportation, etc.?
- If the medical and health care facilities have been affected, what protocols can be taken to ensure the general public has medical care?
- Are escape routes open and accessible during disasters?
- How can information be communicated to responders and the public to protect itself?
- What are your community's warning signals; what do they sound like and what should you should do when you hear them?

Community Non-Pharmaceutical Interventions (NPIs)

Community mitigation helps to slow the spread of the disease when a vaccine is unavailable. This is one of the first steps a community should take. Similar to what was covered about personal NPIs, these common-sense preventatives help a community during times of outbreaks and pandemics.

The CDC explains, "Community NPIs are strategies organizations and community leaders can use to help limit face-to-face contact and ultimately, slow the spread of the infection. These strategies may include making sick-leave policies more flexible in workplace settings, temporarily dismissing schools, avoiding close contact with others, and canceling large public events."

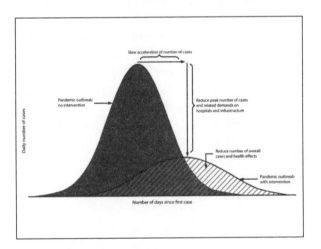

This figure includes two curves, with daily number of influenza cases on the y axis and days since first case on the x axis. One curve shows a pandemic with intervention, and the other curve shows a pandemic without intervention. The curve without intervention begins to slope upward before the curve with intervention and also peaks at a higher point. Goals of community mitigation are shown on the "without intervention" curve and include 1) slow acceleration of number of cases, 2) reduce peak number of cases and related demands on hospitals and infrastructure, and 3) reduce number of cases overall and health effects.

One community NPI that can be implemented early on in an outbreak is reminding children in schools to wash their hands frequently. If children are young, some of these tactics have to be done in a non-scary way.

5 Non-Scary Tips to Teach Your Kids About Germs

1. Germs can make you sick. People can pass colds and other illnesses through germs.
2. Germs are everywhere. They are so small that you cannot see them without a microscope.
3. Cover your mouth and nose with a tissue when you cough or sneeze so you don't pass germs on to others. Throw the tissue in the trash after you use it. Wash your hands the right way to get rid of germs and lower the chance of spreading germs.
4. Wash your hands often with soap and water, especially after you cough or sneeze. Use alcohol-based hand rubs or wipes when soap and water are not available.
5. Don't touch your eyes, nose, or mouth until your hands are clean because germs spread that way. Keeping your hands clean is one of the best ways to keep from getting sick and spreading illness.

Two of the most commonly used community NPIs include:

Social distancing: Creating ways to increase distance between people in settings where people commonly come into close contact with one another. Specific priority settings include schools, workplaces, events, meetings, and other places where people gather.

Closures: Temporarily closing childcare centers, schools, places of worship, sporting events, concerts, festivals, conferences, and other settings where people gather.

Community NPIs, like social distancing and closures, require careful planning and coordination. Public health professionals, planners, and leaders need to work together to help reduce the risk to their organizations and community from respiratory illnesses like pandemic coronavirus or flu. Recommendations include:

- **Connecting.** Collaborate with other professionals, leaders, and administrators in different settings to identify challenges and how they can be overcome in your community.
- **Planning.** When planning for social distancing and closures, seek ideas for what has worked well in the past or could be improved next time. By gathering data, you can identify strategies for making these interventions work smoothly and with as little disruption as possible to your organization or community.
- **Sharing.** Communicate what you have tried and the obstacles you have faced so that other organizations and communities can also benefit from the work you have done.

Multi-Family Living During Pandemics

An epidemic or pandemic outbreak can spread quickly throughout a community—especially for those living in close living situations. The best way to avoid contracting a contagious illness is by limiting your exposure. This is another type of social distancing. Avoid common areas in apartment complexes. If you have to go out near groups of people, wear your personal protective equipment. Consider wearing disposable gloves when checking the mailbox or taking out the trash, as well. Moreover, opt for the stairs instead of using the elevator to get to your apartment or condo. If you must be around others, you need to wear a mask and keep your hands clean with 60% alcohol-based hand sanitizer.

10 Space Savers for Your Preps

1. Baskets and wire bins – Go to discount stores and find large baskets on sale. They can be placed under chairs, benches, and on consoles or above cabinets in the kitchen, if there is extra space.

2. Under bed storage – Under the bed is usually the first place we turn to when our closets run out of space. Plastic containers with lids can be stored under beds. This keeps pets from opening any packages and protects them from the elements. Re-purposing old dresser drawers can also be a solution to under bed storage. And adding wheels to the bottom so they roll out will help you gain easier access.

3. Trundle beds – If your trundle bed is going unused, it's a great place to store your preps. Simply remove the mattress and voilà!

4. Old metal filing cabinets – Consider storing lightweight groups of items such as medical supplies or flashlights and batteries, or even spices in old filing cabinets. It's a great way to organize your preps! Also, if you remove the drawers of the file cabinet and set the cabinet on its backside, it can be used to store brooms, mops, and other household tools..

5. Paper filing boxes – I used this method to store my short-term food supply. We repackaged food in Mylar bags and added them to the filing boxes. I can honestly say this storage methods works, but there are some drawbacks. For one, I would not set heavy items in the boxes. The boxes cannot take much weight and compromises the shape of the box. Stacking the boxes on top of themselves can also be problematic. Still, it is a good storage system and an added benefit is that it's cost effective.

6. Suitcases – For some reason, I have inherited many suitcases over the years. Rather than letting them sit

in a closet, I put them to work. You can even use the luggage tags as labels for the contents.

7. Storage ottomans – I love furniture that serves dual purposes! Storage ottomans are functional in living rooms and will also conceal smaller preps such as your battery supplies, paracord, or books and board games for your off-grid entertainment.

8. Trashcans – Large 35-gallon outdoor trashcans with wheels are also a uniform way to store your gear. Many preppers store their Mylar bagged goods in trash cans for easy access. One could also store their 72-hour emergency supplies in a trashcan for an all-in-one container.

9. Wall space – Wall space is the most under-utilized storage area of a home. Lightweight emergency supplies can be stored on wall shelves. Crates secured to the wall can also make good storage space. Think of collecting many different sized crates to create a crate wall. This would make an amazing storage system.

10. Faux rocks – Hiding your preps camouflaged in faux rocks or statues is another covert way to hide your preps. You can purchase these through garden stores, or make your own. Look online for the right types of clay and design plans.

Pandemic Preparations for the Elderly

The elderly make up a special part of the population which can be prone to illness and chronic health conditions. As people age, their immune systems change, making it harder for their bodies to fight off diseases and infection. Many older adults are also more likely to have underlying health conditions that make it harder to cope with and recover from illness.

This vulnerability can especially put them at risk during times of pandemics. In addition, underlying medical conditions can greatly worsen the course of the illness, probably also as a result of the reduced effectiveness of cell-mediated immunity.

Further, when an aged individual lives in a nursing home facility, this can make them especially prone to catching contagious illnesses more rapidly because of the elderly population living there.

With the elderly more prone to complications that can arise from seasonal influenza, a pandemic version can be devastating, such as we are seeing with COVID-19. The Life Care Center of Kirkland, Washington, had eleven residents dead and others hospitalized, and one health care worker also has been hospitalized. This situation was one of the first outbreaks of COVID-19 to occur in the United States and put into the spotlight the risks associated with the elderly.

Five types of Non-Pharmaceutical Interventions (NPIs) for Elderly Facilities:

- screening visitors and staff who leave and then return to the facility
- isolating symptomatic residents
- placing restrictions on visitors
- modifying work schedules
- precautions taken by staff and visitors to reduce their risk of infection, like washing hands and using protective masks

These prevention efforts not only contribute to care consistency at the facility but also prevent the introduction of viruses by the healthcare workers themselves. Further, employees who come down with illnesses should be given time to recover before returning to work so they no longer represent a threat for introducing the virus.

Elderly living at home

In this COVID-19 outbreak, seniors are especially at risk.

Elderly people should stay at home as much as possible and avoid activities such as traveling by airplane, going to movie theaters, attending family events, shopping at crowded malls, and going to religious services. Make sure you have access to several weeks of medications and supplies in case you need to stay home for prolonged periods of time. When you go out in public, keep away from others who are sick, limit close contact, and wash your hands often.

Here are some ways to prepare:

- Have supplies on hand
- Contact your healthcare provider to ask about obtaining extra necessary medications to have on hand in case there is a pandemic outbreak in your community and you need to stay home for a prolonged period of time.
- If you cannot get extra medications, consider using mail-order for medications.
- Be sure you have over-the-counter medicines and medical supplies (tissues, etc.) to treat fever and other symptoms.
- Have enough household items and groceries on hand so that you will be prepared to stay at home for a period of time.
- Avoid close contact with people who are sick.
- If a pandemic is spreading in your community, take extra measures to put distance between yourself and other people.
- If you feel sick, call your healthcare provider and alert them to your symptoms.
- Stay in touch with others by phone or email. You may need to ask for help from friends, family, neighbors, community health workers, etc. if you become sick.
- Determine who can provide you with care if your caregiver gets sick.
- Take everyday preventive actions:
    - Wash your hands often with soap and water for at least 20 seconds, especially after blowing your

nose, coughing, or sneezing, or having been in a public place.

- If soap and water are not available, use a hand sanitizer that contains at least 60% alcohol.
- To the extent possible, avoid touching high-touch surfaces in public places—elevator buttons, door handles, handrails, handshaking with people, etc. Use a tissue or your sleeve to cover your hand or finger if you must touch something.
- Wash your hands after touching surfaces in public places.
- Avoid touching your face, nose, eyes, etc.
- Clean and disinfect your home to remove germs: practice routine cleaning of frequently touched surfaces (for example: tables, doorknobs, light switches, handles, desks, toilets, faucets, sinks & cell phones).

Elderly in an off-grid environment

Another point to consider is that in a worst-case scenario, if we find ourselves in an off-grid environment without power, the elderly who rely on electricity-dependent medical equipment to stay alive could be placed in a critical, life-threatening situation.

Oftentimes, those that are dependent on medical equipment feel the most vulnerable in the aftermath of an emergency or when the electrical grid is unpredictable. This is especially the case for those whose lives are dependent on a continual source of power. While the elderly population is the first to come to mind in this situation, it is not the only part of the population that could be affected.

Electricity-dependent medical equipment includes:

- Power wheelchairs or mobility devices
- Ventilators

- Oxygen concentrators
- Prescriptions that need to be kept at a certain temperature
- Infusions, intravenous equipment, and feeding equipment
- Chair lifts
- Communication devices
- Nebulizers
- CPAP and other sleep apnea devices
- Suction pumps used by individuals with difficulty swallowing
- Dialysis machines

While this list is not exhaustive, it shows that people of all ages who have a myriad of different afflictions could be affected. Being without some of these devices for as little as a few minutes could be life-threatening.

It is essential to understand that following a large-scale emergency, first responders are inundated with emergency calls and may not be able to reach a person in need in a timely manner. No one wants to see their loved one suffer!

If you are a caretaker, spouse, or family member who has a loved one or friend dependent on electricity-dependent medical equipment, the single most important step one can take is to prepare for the likelihood of being without power. Having a checklist to guide you and help you organize needed supplies and equipment will keep you on track. Moreover, checking this list every six months to ensure all items are accounted for and ready is vital.

For battery-dependent devices:

- Have extra batteries charged and ready to go for durable medical equipment that requires rechargeable batteries. Regularly check backup equipment to ensure it will function appropriately in an emergency.

- Have alternate ways to charge batteries (such as using a USB adapter to charge batteries using a car).
- Make sure all equipment is labeled and that caregivers or family know how to operate it.
- Individuals who use battery-dependent communication devices should have an alternate method for communication readily available.
- Talk to a healthcare provider about non-electricity-dependent alternatives for the equipment listed above or ways to conserve equipment. For example: individuals who use ventilators should keep a resuscitation bag available.
- Individuals who use nebulizers may be able to use inhalers with spacers, which don't require a power supply.
- A doctor may recommend an oxygen user set equipment to reduce flow in order to conserve the supply and extend the life of the system.

As well, the stability of drugs can also be a factor if they need to be refrigerated.

Use an evaporative cooler to keep prescription drugs cool.

According to *Diabetes Management*, "If you do not have an evaporative cooler, for the first day of a power outage, you can keep medications cool in the freezer (although you should unplug it because it will freeze your medications if power is restored). Or you can use an insulated bag or lunchbox with a cold pack, ice, or frozen food from the freezer."[10] A Frio bag would be a valuable investment for keeping medications cold in an off-grid event. This is a reusable evaporative cooler in which the cooling properties come from the evaporation of water. When activated, it keeps its temperature under 78°F for a minimum of two days, even in temperatures of 100°F. This can keep insulin, and many other temperature-sensitive medications, cool and safe. As well, because it is lightweight and compact, it would be perfect for emergency kits and bug-out bags.

Preparing beforehand for times of grid failure is the best way to keep your loved ones safe. As always, make a list of needs and resources, check essential equipment, organize, and plan accordingly. The time will come when you put the plan to action and the more organized it is, the easier the transition into the emergency will be.

Pandemic Considerations for the Homeless

Another key concern when it comes to pandemic planning is the difficulty in caring for those who are homeless. Situational factors such as nutritional vulnerability and compromised immunity, structural factors like close living proximity or inadequate housing in general, and pre-existing health conditions make this population type vulnerable to disease and could lead to further spikes of infection rates within the community.

It may be anticipated that homeless people are at greater risk of becoming sick during a pandemic because:

- Homeless people live in more crowded conditions.
- A widespread outbreak could cause the homeless to panic and migrate from the area and cause further infection to spread to other communities.
- Homeless people often suffer from a variety of chronic and acute conditions which may affect their immune system response.
- They also suffer from addiction and mental illness in rates disparate from the general population and may have problems following advice.
- They may not seek care (and isolation) until they are very sick.
- Social distancing will be difficult to achieve.

Care centers and homeless shelters

When an outbreak occurs, community leaders will begin the process of exploring options for other locations (sometimes called "alternative care sites") that would provide care to people with flu who do not require hospitalization or emergency treatment.

Agencies that provide services to homeless are very diverse. Congregate shelters, apartment-style shelters, voucher programs, and low-income housing programs all have very different ways of providing the homeless with a place to stay. Programs that offer homeless people other services include hygiene centers, employment agencies, drop-in centers, mental health programs, and meal programs. They all provide services to a wide variety of clients and operate under different organizational and funding structures.

Concerns for long-term care

Homeless people enduring mental illnesses may lose continuity of care for an undetermined period of time and may run out of medications due to drug shortages. As well, absenteeism within social service organizations may prevent the homeless population from receiving the care they need.

The role of social services will be paramount in helping to control the spread of a pandemic disease amongst the homeless population. Specifically, these services include surveillance and reporting of diseases to local health authorities, continued case investigation and management, identification and follow-up of close contacts, health risk assessment and communications to the homeless population, liaison with hospitals and other health care system sectors, implementing needed community-based disease control strategies, and providing vaccine and antiviral medication distribution.

School Preparedness

K-12 Schools Emergency Operating Procedures

Schools are currently emphasizing actions such as staying home when sick, appropriately covering coughs and sneezes, cleaning frequently touched surfaces, and washing hands often. This is partly to provide preventative actions and partly to alert the children that they need to do more to protect their health. As well, they will do their part to maintain a clean learning environment; school systems will encourage routinely cleaning frequently touched surfaces (e.g., doorknobs, light switches, countertops) with the cleaners typically used and provide disposable wipes so that commonly used surfaces (e.g., keyboards, desks, remote controls) can be wiped down by students and staff before each use.

Closing schools and teleschooling

During a pandemic emergency, some parents want the schools to close for a given time. School closure can be an effective measure to contain the spread of viruses, but timing and implementation matter. Logistically, it's tricky. That said ,this decision has social, political, and organizational factors that must be considered.

Many schools will try to stay open because closing will affect disadvantaged children more. Free school meals, for example, are an important source of nutrition for many children. Some parents will find it more difficult than others to take time off work to look after their children, and loss of income will hit poorer families harder.

Another consideration is the economic impact closing schools would have on the economy. A study estimated the cost of closing all schools in the US for four weeks at between 10 and 47 billion dollars (0.1–0.3 percent of US GDP). Parents staying home from work comes with significant economic costs. Can you imagine the impact of healthcare workers who have small children and have to stay home to care for them? This makes the school's decision a hard one to make.

The US historical record demonstrates that on multiple occasions, when faced with a contagious crisis that affects children, school dismissal and voluntary absenteeism are common responses. In fact, social distancing measures in the past helped significantly during other historical pandemics:

- One study found that nationwide 18-day school closures in Mexico during the 2009 H1N1 influenza pandemic was associated with a 29% to 37% reduction in flu transmission rates.
- During the much worse 1918 flu pandemic, which killed an estimated 50 million people globally, cities that closed schools and banned public gatherings early during the epidemic had weekly death rates about 50% lower than cities that delayed such closures.

An alternative to closing the school would be to divide the students into smaller groups or utilize internet-based tele-schooling. Implementing online learning or remote schooling is another option, although schools must consider whether all students have access to computers and reliable internet. Schools could send classroom work to students who are under quarantine.

Working in a Pandemic Scare and How to Prepare

Amid a global pandemic, the question of whether to go to work and risk getting ill comes up. It is a given that a severe pandemic may generate extended absences for essential workers that might affect the supply chain. During a severe pandemic, the level of workforce absenteeism may approach 40 percent. To complicate matters, the disease will strike randomly among employees from the boardroom to the mailroom. The loss of critical workers anywhere along the chain from initial receipt to final delivery could cause major disruptions to the entire process.

Even if you are practicing proper hand washing, covering your coughs and sneezes, and cleaning frequently touched surfaces, the fear is still there. Workplaces may need to take a look and make some revisions to their workplace preparations.

6 Workplace Must-Haves During a Pandemic Scare

Implementing disciplined personal hygiene and social distancing strategies in the workplace may reduce potential worker absenteeism for illness and other related reasons. Businesses may consider stockpiling these items:

1. Soap
2. Tissues
3. Hand sanitizer
4. Medications
5. Cleaning supplies
6. Bulk quantities of recommended personal protective equipment: eye protection, facemasks, gloves

When stockpiling items, be aware of each product's shelf life and storage conditions (i.e., avoid areas that are damp or have temperature extremes) and incorporate product rotation (i.e., consume oldest supplies first) into your stockpile management program.

10 Tips for workplaces (from the CDC)

Having a plan in place is essential. Coordinate your planning activities with local public health officials and key community partners and stakeholders to help maintain essential services.

1. **Promote the daily practice of everyday preventive actions at all times.** Stay home if you are sick for at least 24 hours after you no longer have a fever or signs of

a fever without use of fever-reducing medicines. Cover your coughs and sneezes with a tissue, wash your hands often using soap and water for 20 seconds or use 60% alcohol-based hand sanitizer, clean frequently touched surfaces and objects.

2. **Provide prevention supplies in your workplace.** Have supplies on hand for workers, such as soap, hand sanitizer with at least 60% alcohol, tissues, trash baskets, and disposable facemasks. Plan to have extra supplies on hand during a pandemic. Note: Disposable facemasks should be kept on-site and used only when someone becomes sick at the workplace. Those who become sick should be given a clean disposable facemask to wear until they can leave.

3. **Plan for worker absences.** Develop flexible pandemic flu attendance and sick-leave policies. Workers may need to stay home when they are sick, caring for a sick household member, or caring for their children in the event of school dismissals. Identify critical job functions and positions, and plan for alternative coverage by cross-training staff (similar to planning for holiday staffing).

4. **Develop a method for monitoring and tracking virus-related worker absences.** Understand your usual absenteeism patterns at each worksite. Determine what level of absenteeism will disrupt day-to-day operations. If worker absenteeism increases to disruptive levels, some workplaces may need to consider temporarily reducing on-site operations and services.

5. **Identify space that can be used to separate sick people (if possible).** Designate a space for people who may become sick and cannot leave the workplace immediately. If possible, designate a nearby separate bathroom just for sick people. Develop a plan for cleaning the room daily. Find ways to increase space between people to at least 3 feet or limit face-to-face contact

between workers and those who come to the workplace. Several ways to do this include offering workers the option to telework, creating reduced or staggered work schedules, spacing workers farther apart, and postponing non-essential meetings and travel.

6. **Develop a risk-assessment and risk-management process for your workplace.** Work closely with local public health officials to develop a contingency plan if assessing and managing risks among workers and those who come to your workplace is needed (for example, conducting health screenings for symptoms). Note: Your Human Resources Manager may want to review the current Employee Assistance Program (EAP) to ensure workers will have access to needed emotional and mental health services during and after a pandemic.

7. **Review your process for planning workplace events.** Identify actions to take if you need to temporarily postpone or cancel events.

8. **Plan ways to continue essential services if on-site operations are reduced temporarily.** Provide web and mobile-based communication and services, if possible. Increase the use of email, conference calls, video conferencing, and web-based seminars.

9. **Be familiar with your local board of education's pandemic plans.** Local public health officials may recommend schools be dismissed for up to 2 weeks until they have time to gather information about how fast the pandemic is spreading in your community. Workers with children may need the flexibility to work from home.

10. **Encourage workers to plan for alternative childcare arrangements now.**

Travel Bans

Travel bans can also become an issue when a pandemic is circulating the globe. In regards to the COVID-19 outbreak, as of March 11, the US has restricted travel from China and the European Union. However, as the spread of the virus continues, given what has taken place in other countries, we could expect domestic travel bans that will restrict movement from city to city and perhaps from home to home, should the government take worst case scenario precautions.

If a person who is traveling finds themselves in an epicenter of an outbreak, they should expect the following messages from an airline:

- "You should return to your homes or places of accommodation and we will send you more information when it is available,"
- "We are working with authorities in order to reschedule the flight for tomorrow,"
- "As you had a previously confirmed seat/s on the aircraft this evening, your seat is confirmed for the next flight which we anticipate will depart on (a specific date),"
- "We know that this unexpected delay will cause stress and inconvenience, which we regret."

These delays have the potential to last days or weeks depending on the severity of the outbreak and, in order to beat the panic, action on your part must be taken quickly.

When you start noticing that the situation you are is wrong, it is time to start acting. One of the first things you can do is to install the airline app on your phone. This will provide you with quick access to information and essential website links that will give flight status information and where you can book an alternative flight. Here are five additional immediate actions to take.

1. Book a hotel right away. In addition, once you know that you're getting bumped from a flight, an immediate

call to a hotel is suggested. When a hotel knows there are travel troubles, they can hike the price of a stay.

2. Stay in contact with your airline. Tied up phone lines and a long queue at the counter will most likely keep you from talking with a live airline representative.

3. Have extra money. Carrying extra money with you is essential in times such as these. While a credit is also handy, in emergency situations, cash may be the king! Cash will allow you to purchase food, transportation, and necessary items during unexpected travel bans or delays. Further, if you are stranded and given a hotel voucher, sometimes the hotels are filled to capacity and there are no other rooms. You may have to find a room in a different hotel. Plus, cash will help you buy food or some water if you find yourself hungry or thirsty. Likewise, inform your credit card company about the situation. If you booked with a credit card, some card companies could reimburse your meals and lodging during these times.

4. Have a carry-all bag with critical items. There may be no telling how long you'll be kept inside your terminal or asked to come back at a later date. With that, the following items are the most needed: high protein snacks, an empty water bottle, a change of clothes, a warm sweatshirt, toothpaste and toothbrush, headphones, earplugs, phone charger, and a book. Having an empty water bottle will save you so much money because you can fill the bottle up from a water fountain. Bottled water can be pricey at airports.

5. Choose your territory. If you cannot find additional lodging, it's time to choose a spot in the airport. Look for some space that no one is holding up and get there as fast as you can and set up your domain. If you are held up for more than just a few hours, you better be in a place you can call yours! Get all your baggage and

secure the area and snuggle up for the long haul—that travel pillow will definitely come in handy!

BONUS TIP: Take this time to practice your situational awareness skills. This is perhaps the most important thing you can do while traveling, and it applies no matter your destination, stranded or not.

It should be mentioned that you should always pay attention to your surroundings and stay alert. Keep your head up, watch what is going on around you, and acknowledge people. Project a strong and aware demeanor.

Health screenings and checkpoints

When you finally get a chance to evacuate the viral hot zone, expect extremely long lines and wait times for public health screenings and checkpoints. As well, at the checkpoints, health officials may check for symptoms and/or provide you with a questionnaire that will ask passengers if they have experienced symptoms such as a cough or fever. In addition, the survey will also ask if travelers had visited the area where the outbreak began.

At the heath screening, passengers may go through thermal scanners that will take their body temperatures. Those with fevers will then undergo further evaluation.

- If you have fever, cough, or trouble breathing: the health officials at the airport will evaluate you for illness. You will be taken to a medical facility for further evaluation and care. You may not be able to complete your travel itinerary.
- If you do not have symptoms: You will be allowed to reach your final destination. After arrival at your final destination, you will be asked to monitor your health for a period of how long the incubation period for the illness lasts. You will receive a health information card

that tells you what symptoms to look for and what to do if you develop symptoms. During that time, you should stay home and limit interactions with others as much as possible. Your state or local health department will contact you for further follow-up.

If there is exposure at an airport

What if a passenger was sick on your flight? What if that person was later diagnosed with a serious infectious disease and was contagious during your flight? Are you at risk? If you were exposed, how do you protect yourself?

Although the risk of getting a contagious disease on an airplane is low, public health officers sometimes need to find and alert travelers who may have been exposed to a sick passenger on a flight. The search for these travelers is known as a contact investigation. A contact investigation or health screening is one of the ways to protect the health of people exposed to an illness during travel and to protect their communities from contagious diseases that are just a flight away.

Protecting travelers' health from airport to community (excerpted from the CDC)

A contact investigation often starts with a phone call to a CDC Quarantine Station located at a US international airport. The caller is a public health official who informs CDC about a recent air traveler diagnosed with a specific contagious disease. Sometimes CDC is notified about a sick traveler while the plane is still in the air or shortly after the plane has landed. However, in most cases CDC is notified when a sick traveler seeks treatment at a medical facility. These notifications can be made days, weeks, or even months after the travel. This sick traveler is now referred to as the "index patient."

The caller notifies CDC because other passengers on the arriving international flight or connecting domestic flights may have been exposed and need to be notified. Or an international partner calls CDC about exposed US passengers on overseas flights. The passengers exposed to the index patient are called "contacts."

CDC is responsible for coordinating contact investigations of illness exposures on arriving international flights or flights between states. A single infected traveler can trigger more than one contact investigation if the traveler takes connecting flights to reach a US destination.

A person can be contagious without showing any symptoms while the disease is developing (incubating) in the body. Quarantine public health officers must determine whether the index patient was contagious during a flight. Their decision is based on the disease, history of symptoms, and date of the flight.

Starting the contact investigation

If the index patient was contagious during the flight, passengers seated nearby may have been exposed to the disease. CDC will start a contact investigation to find these passengers.

CDC requests the flight manifest for passengers seated near the index patient. The flight manifest is a document that contains passengers' names, seat numbers, and contact information. CDC guards the privacy of passengers by keeping this information secure.

Note: This is a good reminder to make sure you give the correct contact information to the airlines when you book your flight! Also, remember to update your frequent flyer program contact information.

How Communities Can Move Forward After a Pandemic Ends

Communities who provided good public containment efforts should be proud that they took the health concerns seriously and may have saved many lives as a result. When the pandemic is nearing a close, community leaders should focus their efforts on rebuilding the community as well as safeguarding them from future outbreaks. The WHO provides four essential suggestions on how to help communities achieve this.

1. Ask essential services to develop recovery plans for their service or organization.
2. Define responsibilities for social, psychological, and practical support to affected families and companies. If needed, organize training and education for personnel involved.
3. Assess how existing community groups (religious groups/churches, sports groups) can contribute to rebuilding the society. Identify contact persons within these groups.
4. Consider whether recovery after a pandemic needs financial support from the government. If so, develop criteria for financial support and seek ways to ensure availability of funds.

In order for a community and/or country to begin thriving as it once had, questions should be raised by local, state, and federal leaders when the pandemic is nearing an end. Some of these questions are:

- Is there a plan in place to ensure the quick revitalization of the country after a pandemic?
- Do essential services have recovery plans?
- Who should be responsible to provide social and psychological support to affected families and companies?
- Is there a mechanism in place to assess economic losses and to provide financial support to affected groups?

Conclusion

Preventing the transmission of an illness rests in the hands of not only the individual, but the community as well. Proper planning and prevention play a key role in preparing for a pandemic. There is a lot to be said for preventative measures.

Communities as a whole should take the necessary steps to be prepared for potential pandemic challenges before a threat exists. Understand that large congregation areas, e.g., malls, schools, airports, and grocery stores, also pose a hazard to spreading the pandemic more quickly. Breakdowns in communications, supply chains, payroll service issues, transportation, and healthcare staff shortages should be anticipated when preparing for a pandemic.

It doesn't take much, in general, for a virus to go from being worrisome to being extremely worrisome. But anticipating the needs of the community and issues that may arise is the first step to a happy, safe, and healthy community.

CHAPTER 7

What Will Our Future Look Like?

After a pandemic wave is over, it can be expected that there could be great loss and the surviving population could be affected in a variety of ways. In the event of a long-term, widely spread pandemic event, many may have lost friends or relatives, suffer from fatigue, or have financial losses as a result of the interruption of business.

The question remains, is it possible to eradicate a pandemic disease? As the WHO simply states, this is "difficult and rarely achieved." So how does a pandemic most likely end?

Here are five theories:

1. One possibility is that cases of the disease will start decreasing when enough people develop immunity, either through infection or with the help of a vaccination.
2. Another possible scenario is that the virus will continue to circulate and establish itself as a common respiratory virus.
3. A pandemic virus can mutate either in a more destructive manner or in a positive way, making it more difficult for the virus to infect people.
4. A pandemic is usually multi-phasic. It is important not to forget that another wave may lie ahead. To circumvent this, staying ever vigilant and continuing preparedness strategies is of the essence.

5. It can take months or years for a vaccine to become available; therefore, this could become a new normal.

There are a lot of unknowns when it comes to a pandemic, but here is what we know: the world has been hit time and time again with diseases that span the globe killing many in its wake, but somehow we are still here. In the developed world, we have been able to hold off the takeover of these pandemic diseases using vaccines, antibiotics, and the natural eradication of certain diseases.

When you reach the end phases of a pandemic, the world as you know it has permanently changed. The "system" will no longer work in the same way it had before the event. This begs the question of what a post-pandemic world would look like.

A Post-Pandemic World

Many wonder what our future will look like after this pandemic and if there will be long-term ramifications as a result of this world event.

The world's goal will be not only to contain the outbreaks, but also to keep the economy and systems going as best as possible, under the circumstances.

Despite our strides in medical technology and modern living, significant gaps and challenges will always exist with global pandemics. Depending how long lasting this pandemic is, it could have the capacity to change the way you engage in your community and even cause long-term shortages to household staples. Are you prepared for a world without antibiotics?

In a post-pandemic world, our lives may have changed permanently.

- The economic damage is already occurring through multiple channels, including short-term fiscal shocks, and will likely continue with longer-term negative shocks to economic growth.

- There could be short or long-term behavioral changes, including people not wanting to go out in public out of fear of contracting a disease. Some pandemic mitigation measures can cause significant social and economic disruption. Political stressors could also effect change.
- On an individual level, further paranoia could occur during a post-pandemic life when one comes down with a seasonal illness.
- In countries with weak institutions and legacies of political instability, pandemics can increase political stresses and tensions.
- Measures such as quarantines may spark violence, looting, and tension between states and citizens due to lack of response, supply shortages, or overall panic over the situation. These sorts of tensions do not quickly dissipate.
- From a health standpoint, there may be long-term health consequences as a result of contracting the pandemic illness or shortages of healthcare workers as a result of illness or death.

But there could be some good that that could come out of a pandemic:

- Modern technology may play a larger role in keeping parts of the fragile system going. Adapting to a pandemic and causing schools and businesses to close creates a different technical environment. We could be ordering groceries online more, which makes more time to spend with the family. Kids are staying home and teleschooling and parents have found new ways to stay home and work remotely. This provides the school and work environments the time they need to get ready and open their doors again.

- A pandemic event when families stay in their homes for weeks or months could cause a heightened demand on the internet, thus causing slow load times. This could be an opportunity for parents to introduce other activities besides video games and social media.
- If families are spending more time in a post-pandemic world, they can learn from each other. If Dad does the house repairs, and Mom is the gardener, why not teach those skills to the children? That way, they can come out of this situation with a skill set and an ability to be more self-reliant so they do not repeat history.
- Our country may shift focus from outsourcing and getting goods from other countries to bringing jobs and goods back to the US. This could create a rebirth in the economy and help stabilize the economy.
- Businesses that had to close their doors during the pandemic may have adapted and found a way to generate income online, thus opening new doors to customers.
- Consider for a moment the change a pandemic such as this could have on our healthcare system. Having an initial appointment online rather than waiting in a doctor's office or hospital could help doctors' offices be more efficient in patient care and cut down on seasonal illnesses.

Learning from the Past

A pandemic can last for several months, if not years, and the impact on individuals, households, and communities could be long felt. While many imagine a bleak existence following a pandemic, we need only look to our past to remember that pandemics come and go and we as humans endure and survive.

A hundred years ago, our world was in a deadly battle against another virus, the Spanish Flu. Somehow there were parts of the world untouched by this deadly pathogen. How did these communities escape when everywhere around them was affected?

In a study of seven communities unaffected by the Spanish Flu, they found something startling. The communities were: the rural farming village of Fletcher, in northern Vermont; Gunnison, Colorado, a remote town in the Rocky Mountains; Princeton University in New Jersey; Bryn Mawr College in Pennsylvania; the Western Pennsylvania Institution for the Blind in Pittsburgh; and the Trudeau Tuberculosis Sanatorium in Saranac Lake, New York.

> . . . one of the great strengths of our study is the diversity of our 7 communities. Consequently, we believe that important historical lessons can and should be extracted from a careful and close examination of the communities profiled in this study.

In an interview with the BBC,[11] Markal explains:

> "These communities basically shut themselves down," explains Howard Markel, an epidemiological historian at the University of Michigan who was one of the authors of the study. "No one came in and no one came out. Schools were closed and there were no public gatherings. We came up with the term 'protective sequestration', where a defined and healthy group of people are shielded from the risk of infection from outsiders."

While these findings have helped experts in the health field around the world make necessary recommendations to better prepare for pandemics, ultimately they show that communities can survive when plagues are present.

In that intriguing study of the seven influenza escape communities, Howard Markal provides stunning insight into what future pandemic survival may grapple with. In his haunting words on what we could likely see in the recovery phase of a pandemic, "What is most troubling about this phase is that although it can lead to retrospection and action in terms of preparedness for subsequent epidemic events, all too often it leads to complacency or even outright amnesia about the event."

Personal Preparedness

Keeping those crucial words on complacency to heart, we must never stop preparing.

As pandemics are ever evolving, so should you be ever evolving in order to survive them. Adapting to a situation is the cornerstone for survival. Simply put, staying fluid helps you stay open to change in an ever-changing situation. Our communities should also be fluid.

Supply lines and necessary items for household living may still be in high demand, so it is important to anticipate this struggle to have future supplies in place. Either learn to adapt or find alternatives.

When public health officials determine the pandemic has ended in your community, take time to improve your household's emergency plan. Keep a list of everything you needed and what you could have done to make things run more efficiently and start preparing for the next wave or next emergency.

Our modern way of life is not promised. The infrastructures is fragile and, as we have mentioned, one event has the capacity to level it. One of the most important things to do is to train your mind to handle these hardships. As the world at large faces an uncertain future in regard to pandemics, the readiness factor relies on each of us. Continue stocking up on foods that have the capacity to last long, investing in freeze-dried foods to be ready for the next disaster, and invest in seeds for long-term food security. Consider looking into more off-grid methods and tools that can add convenience during difficult times. One example is the Sun Oven. These nifty contraptions can be used to cook, pasteurize water, can food, dehydrate foods, warm or dry clothes, refrigerate foods during cold weather, and even make ghee! Or try your hand at hydroponics! The point is to start looking into a different way of life.

Staying Strong in the Most Difficult of Times

The mind is a very powerful muscle in the body. In fact, it's the strongest muscle, and it has the capacity to make or break you. It can either propel you through a challenge or paralyze you into inaction. Therefore, having control over the mind gives you the wherewithal you need to withstand biological and emotional stressors during disasters or life events, as well as better adapt to the situation at hand. In fact, Navy SEALS use this technique in their training, which is why they are always cool and collected when in dangerous environments.

If the mind is untrained, it can easily go to a place of hopelessness and negativity where eventually a person gives up altogether. If you're caught in a situation in which you feel powerless, there are two scenarios that could play out: 1.) You can imagine yourself as a hero, figuring a way through the problem, or 2.) You can imagine yourself as a victim, suffering and waiting for rescue. Which would you choose? (The answer is that you are going to figure a way out and survive!) Remember, it's all in your attitude!

How to be resilient

Being resilient does not mean that a person doesn't experience difficulties or distress. In fact, developing resilience is likely to involve considerable emotional distress. It is what gives people the ability to come back from disappointment and failure stronger and more determined than ever.

Resilience is not a trait or characteristic that you either have or don't have. It is a learned ability, one that can be learned and built and developed by anyone. Resilience relies on different skills and draws on various sources of help, including rational thinking skills, physical and mental health, and your relationships with those around you. Resilient people not only survive and bounce back after a setback, but they also come back stronger and wiser. People who are highly resilient are excellent at finding the silver lining in any situation. They excel in finding the lesson each negative experience has taught them and applying what they learned in future endeavors.

One principle you must keep in mind when dealing with emergencies is that change is inevitable. Change is the one true constant in this universe, yet it is something we tend to stress about and avoid altogether. Many do not handle stress well because they are unprepared to deal with what has been thrown at them. They are resistant to change. This rigidity will only hinder them from finding solutions. Disasters bring change and a lot of it. An aspect of mental preparedness, therefore, is learning to be more fluid and respectful of change in your day-to-day life. This ease in movement and acceptance of change will help you adapt more quickly to all situations. The more flexible you learn to be, the more adaptable you will be in an emergency.

We have all heard that practice makes perfect. One way to be mentally prepared for situations of extreme stress, therefore, is to hold rehearsal drills. Consistent practice will turn your life-saving plans into muscle memory. This rehearse-to-be-ready concept is how many emergency personnel and even athletes train to condition their mind and body. This could make all the difference when stress is sending your neurotransmitters out of whack. Even implementing stress relief techniques when responding to daily stress helps. The daily "minor disasters" give valuable insight into your mental and physical reaction to stressors, allowing you to know how you best perform under pressure.

Any pandemic has the capacity to kill large groups of our population and turn the world upside down in its wrath, but if we learn the lessons of preparing for longer-term emergencies, isolating, quarantining, and locking down homes or communities, their unrelenting nature will diminish. Because we do not fully understand the nature of viruses, we will always be one step behind them. All we can do is prepare the best we can and use the lessons we learn from historic pandemics as guides for what to do and what not to do.

With COVID-19, the time has come for us to open our eyes and to stop being complacent. In each of our lives we will face one emergency after another. Sometimes these emergencies are minor, and sometimes they are living nightmares. But if you can plan for them and prepare for what you might need, they can be less burdensome.

Endnotes

1   "WHO Director-General's Opening Remarks at the Media Briefing on COVID-19 - 2 March 2020." World Health Organization. Accessed March 12, 2020. https://www.who.int/dg/speeches/detail/who-director-general-s-opening-remarks-at-the-media-briefing-on-covid-19---2-march-2020.

2   Wang, Dawei. "Clinical Characteristics of Patients with 2019 Novel Coronavirus (2019-NCoV)–Infected Pneumonia in Wuhan, China." JAMA, February 7, 2020. https://jamanetwork.com/journals/jama/fullarticle/2761044.

3   "Nieman Guide to Covering Pandemic Flu: The Science: How Flu Viruses Change." Nieman Guide to Covering Pandemic Flu | The Science | How Flu Viruses Change. Accessed March 12, 2020. https://nieman.harvard.edu/wp-content/uploads/pod-assets/microsites/NiemanGuideToCoveringPandemicFlu/TheScience/HowFluVirusesChange.aspx.html.

4   "ACE2 Shedding and Furin Abundance in Target Organs May Influence the Efficiency of SARS-CoV-2 Entry." ChinaXiv.org. Accessed March 12, 2020. http://www.chinaxiv.org/abs/202002.00082.

5   "ACE2 Shedding and Furin Abundance in Target Organs May Influence the Efficiency of SARS-CoV-2 Entry." ChinaXiv.org. Accessed March 12, 2020. http://www.chinaxiv.org/abs/202002.00082.

6   www.cdc.gov/flu/pandemic-resources/pdf/pandemic-influenza-implementation.pdf, accessed March 12, 2020

7   "Transcript for CDC Telebriefing: CDC Update on Novel Coronavirus." *Transcript for CDC Telebriefing: CDC Update on Novel Coronavirus*, February 5, 2020. https://www.cdc.gov/media/releases/2020/t0205-coronavirus-update.html.

8   "When and How to Wash Your Hands." Centers for Disease Control and Prevention. Centers for Disease Control and Prevention, October 3, 2019. https://www.cdc.gov/handwashing/when-how-handwashing.html.

9   Guidance on Preparing Workplaces for an Influenza Pandemic. Accessed March 13, 2020. https://www.osha.gov/Publications/influenza_pandemic.html#steps_employers_can_take.

10   Katzki, Lisa, and Bsn. "Disaster Preparedness and Diabetes - How to Manage Your Diabetes: Diabetes Self." Management. Diabetes Self Management, July 22, 2016. https://www.diabetesselfmanagement.com/managing-diabetes/general-health-issues/disaster-preparedness-diabetes/.

11   Gray, Richard. "The Places That Escaped the Spanish Flu." BBC Future. BBC, October 24, 2018. https://www.bbc.com/future/article/20181023-the-places-that-escaped-the-spanish-flu.

Full Pandemic Supply List

ITEMS TO FIND THE DOLLAR STORE

- Paper plates and plastic utensils
- Zip-loc storage bags
- Water (1 gallon per day)
- Salt and pepper
- Spices and condiments
- Cereal
- Peanut butter
- Juice per family member
- Canned vegetables and fruit
- Boxed dinners (macaroni and cheese, hamburger helper, etc.)
- Cans of meat per family member (tuna, salmon, chicken, Spam, etc.)
- Canned soup or stew
- Non-perishable items (saltine crackers, graham crackers, oatmeal, granola bars, pasta, etc.)
- Hand-operated can opener
- First aid items such as antibiotic ointment, band-aids, gauze, elastic bandages, Tylenol
- Toilet paper and paper towels
- Feminine needs
- Cigarette lighters and/or matches
- Candles
- Canning jars
- Multi-vitamins
- Flashlights
- Batteries
- Weatherproof tape
- Trash bags
- Soap
- Cleaning sponges
- Bleach
- Toothpaste/toothbrush

FOOD

- Canned fruits, vegetables, meats, and soups
- Dried legumes
- Crackers
- Nuts
- Pasta sauce
- Pasta
- Peanut butter
- Flour
- Whole grains – Steel-cut oats, bulgur, Whole-grain couscous
- Seasonings (salt, pepper, cinnamon, favorite spice combinations, bouillon cubes or granules)
- Sugar
- Baking staples – baking powder, baking soda, yeast, vinegar)
- Honey
- Unsweetened cocoa powder
- Jell-O or pudding mix
- Plant based oil

- Cereals
- Seeds for eating or sprouting
- Popcorn
- Instant potato flakes
- Rice
- Packaged meals (hamburger helper, macaroni and cheese, etc.)
- Protein bars
- Protein powder
- Jerky and air-dried beef
- Dehydrated meat
- Bone broth
- Protein pancakes or waffles

- Dried milk
- Fresh fruits – citrus fruits, apples, berries, bananas
- Fresh vegetables – green leafy vegetables, broccoli, carrots, beets, onions, etc.
- Potatoes
- Coffee, teas, fruit juices, drink mixes
- Crisco (can use as makeshift emergency candles, fire starters, etc.)
- Freeze-dried meats, vegetables, fruits, and eggs
- Pet food

WATER

- Cases of bottled water
- High quality filtration system (Berkey water filter, Kataydyn Water Filter, etc.)

- Purification tablets
- Bleach (for purifying water and for sanitation needs)

HYGEINE

- Liquid antibacterial hand soap
- Disposable hand wipes
- Antibacterial hand sanitizer
- Feminine hygiene items – one months worth

- Extra baby needs (diapers, wipes, pacifiers, bottles, medicine, etc.) – in quantity
- Exam gloves
- Tissues

SANITATION

- Disinfectant – bleach, Lysol spray
- Durable cleaning gloves
- Heavy-duty gallon sized trash bags

- Clorox wipes
- Paper towels
- Toilet paper
- Hand wipes

NATURAL CARE*

- Multivitamins
- Vitamin A, B, C, D, E, Zinc
- Ginger
- Garlic
- Ginseng

- Oregano oil
- Colloidal silver
- Tinctures to boost immune system

- Immune boosting herbal teas – echinacea, rosehip, ginger, hibiscus, rooibos, sage, lemon balm
- Probiotics
- Spirulina
- Apple cider vinegar (with mother)
- Aloe vera
- Essential oils that have antimicrobial action will also help fight germs. Herbs such as basil, cassia, cinnamon, eucalyptus, frankincense, lemon, lemongrass, marjoram, Melaleuca, myrrh, oregano, four thieves oil, and thyme.

*Natural remedies do not cure pandemic illnesses but give needed support to the immune system.

PERSONAL PROTECTIVE EQUIMENT

- Disposable gown
- Eye goggles or protective eyewear
- Disposable surgical gloves
- N95 respirator
- Hand sanitizer
- Tyvek protective suit rated to guard against biological hazards

OVER-THE-COUNTER PRODUCTS

- Aspirin or non-aspirin pain reliever (for adults and children)
- Rubbing alcohol
- Betadine
- Stool softener
- Electrolyte powder
- Cold/flu medications
- Expectorant/decongestants
- Topical decongestants
- Short-acting beta agonist inhalers
- Glucose Tablets

PRESCRIPTION MEDICATIONS

- Essential prescription medications you are dependent on – a 1-month supply, if possible
- Antibiotics – this does not protect against viral

epidemics but can help in a long-term emergency to guard against bacterial infections.
- Tamiflu

ESSENTIAL MEDICAL TOOLS - (for extended emergency planning)

- Trauma shears
- Penlight or small flashlight
- Scalpel with extra blades
- Cotton balls
- Stethoscope
- Irrigation syringe
- Tweezers
- Thermometer
- Thermometer

WOUND CARE (for extended emergency planning)

- Disinfectant (Betadine, isopropyl alcohol, iodine, hydrogen peroxide, etc.) member
- Band-aids
- Antibiotic ointment
- Instant cold and hot packs
- Ace bandages
- Non- stick gauze pads in assorted sizes (3×3 and 4×4)
- Sterile roller bandages
- Surgical sponges
- Adhesive tape or duct tape
- Steri-strips
- Moleskin
- Respirator masks
- CPR micro shield
- Suture kit
- QuikClot® compression bandages
- Tourniquet
- Thermal Mylar blanket
- Antibiotics

SICK ROOM ITEMS:

- Tyvek protective suit and shoe covers
- Plastic sheeting
- Bed with linens, pillow and blanket
- Small wastebasket or a bucket lined with a plastic garbage bag.
- Gallon-sized zip-loc bags
- Pitcher or large bottle for water
- Large plastic dishpan
- A portable toilet and human waste bags
- Clipboard with paper and a pen for writing in the daily log.
- Clock
- Hand crank or battery-powered radio
- Good source of light
- Flashlight with extra batteries
- A clothing hamper or a garbage can lined with a plastic garbage bag can be used to collect soiled clothing and bedding items before they are washed.
- A bell or a noisemaker to call for assistance.
- Thermometer
- Tissues
- Hand wipes or a waterless hand sanitizer
- Bleach or disinfectant
- Air disinfectants
- Antibacterial soap
- Cotton balls
- Rubbing alcohol, disinfectant or bleach
- Measuring cup capable of holding 8 ounces or 250 ml
- Over-the-counter medications for use in the sick room
- Protective eye gear
- Protective clothing
- Disposable aprons or smocks (at least 2 cases)
- Duct tape for sealing off doorways and vents
- Latex household disposable cleaning gloves
- Disposable nitrile gloves (2-3 boxes)
- Garbage bags
- Trash can

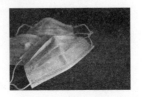

- N95 masks or N100 respirator masks
- Disposable faceshield
- Vaporizers
- Vaporizer solution
- Humidifiers – warm air / cool air
- Biohazard waste containers
- Water containers
- HEPA air purifier / filters
- Labels
- Sharpie markers

CRITIAL ITEMS FOR TRAVELING

- Snacks
- Empty water bottle
- Change of clothes
- Warm sweatshirt
- Travel pillow
- Toothpaste and toothbrush
- Earphones
- Earplugs
- Phone charger

PERSONAL

- Money
- Hand crank or battery-powered radio
- Flashlight with extra batteries
- Headlamps
- Gas lanterns
- Matches/lighter

INFORMATION AND RECORDS

- Blood type
- Immunization / vaccination record
- Medical history
- Medications, OTC's, herbals
- Allergies
- Health conditions
- Co-morbidities / disease states
- Lifestyle – smoking / tobacco use, alcohol use, exercise
- Information – Names, Phone numbers,
- Addresses
- Family members
- Caregivers
- Physicians
- Insurance / 3rd party coverage
- Financial status / payment ability